THE
4-WEEK
INSOMNIA
WORKBOOK

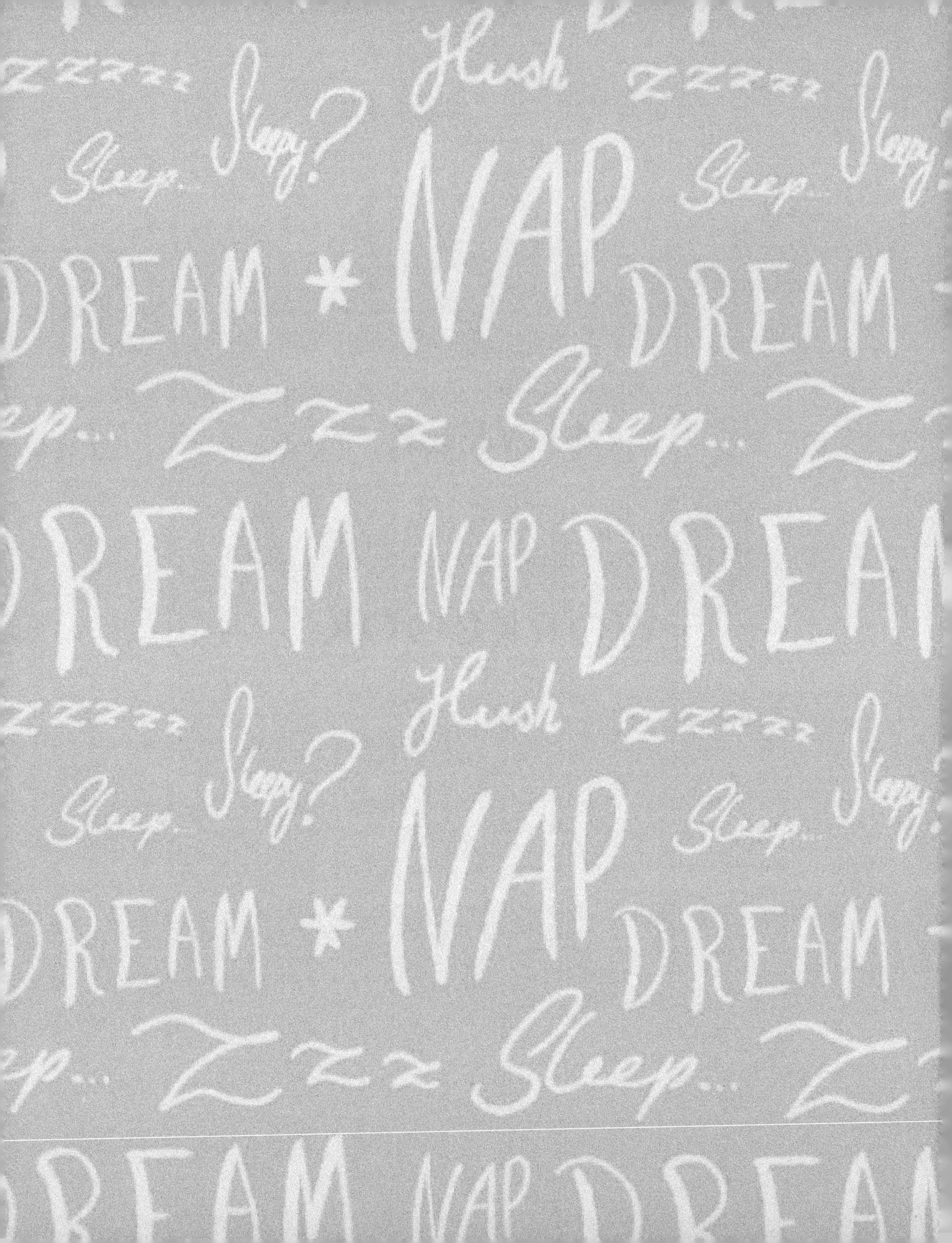

Hush
Zzzzzz
Sleepy?
Sleep...
NAP
DREAM
Zzz

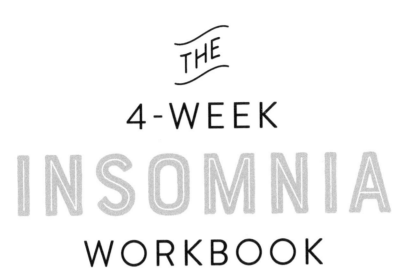

THE
4-WEEK
INSOMNIA
WORKBOOK

A DRUG-FREE PROGRAM

to Build Healthy Habits and Achieve Restful Sleep

Sara Dittoe Barrett, PhD

ALTHEA
PRESS

For general information on our other products and services or to obtain technical support, please contact our Customer Care Department within the U.S. at (866) 744-2665, or outside the U.S. at (510) 253-0500.

Althea Press publishes its books in a variety of electronic and print formats. Some content that appears in print may not be available in electronic books, and vice versa.

Interior and Cover Designer: Peatra Jariya
Editor: Nana K. Twumasi
Production Editor: Erum Khan
Cover: Nesser3321/ iStock
Author photo © Chad Leverenz

ISBN: Print 978-1-64152-469-8 | eBook 978-1-64152-470-4

FOR PAIGE

AND PATRICK,

WHO HAVE ALWAYS BEEN WORTH

THE SLEEPLESS NIGHTS.

CONTENTS

INTRODUCTION

THERE ARE TWO DISTINCT PERIODS IN MY LIFE when I suffered from chronic insomnia. The first was when I was a teenager in high school, and it lasted for about two years. I had several bad habits that contributed to many sleepless nights. I consistently got less sleep than I needed during the week because of how early I had to wake up, and homework and after-school activities kept me up late. I mistakenly thought I could repay this sleep debt by sleeping in late on weekends or taking naps. These bad habits led to my lying awake on Sunday nights, fretting about how tired and miserable I would be on Monday morning. I complained often about my lack of sleep and inability to fall asleep. I clearly remember the frustration, stress, worry, and misery I felt about sleep.

The second bout of insomnia occurred after the birth of my first child. This time, the lack of sleep was more pronounced. My daughter was not one of those magical babies who would sleep through the night. In fact, she did not sleep much at all, and when she did, it was during the day. And at that point in my life, I was staring into the blue light of a screen every night, either looking at the video monitor to see if the baby was okay or at multiple other devices as I fed the baby and watched Netflix, read, or googled phrases like "Does sleep deprivation cause brain damage?" I read five books on how to get my daughter to sleep on my schedule. I was unable to accept her fragmented, unpredictable sleep, and even more unable to accept my own sleep deprivation. My husband was also not sleeping as much, often taking the early morning baby shift. I worried about how no one in our house was sleeping well. When I did sleep, it was often short and shallow because I had significant anxiety and worried about the baby often, checking on her frequently at night. Eventually my daughter did start sleeping through the night. But by that point, my brain seemed trained to be awake, alert, and hypervigilant in the middle of the night. I am more of a night owl than a morning person, so my natural tendency to work late into the evening to get things done did not match my daughter's happy, bright-eyed 5 a.m. wake-ups that lasted for years. My brain, my natural rhythms, and my sleep and work habits were all working against my getting enough good, solid sleep.

Luckily, the insomnia did not last forever. But it didn't have anything to do with luck. I started practicing good sleep hygiene. I used the tools I now teach my clients to retrain my brain that nighttime and bed were for sleeping. I used mindfulness and created a wind-down routine that improved the quality of my sleep. I still have periods of disrupted sleep, especially when my stress level is high, but I struggle with insomnia less and know what to do to work with it.

You are likely reading this because you are currently battling with insomnia. I have been there, and I am excited that you have picked up this book. The strategies described here are the best that cognitive behavioral therapy (CBT) has to offer. They are backed by a large amount of scientific research, and the program itself has enough flexibility that you can tailor it to your individual needs. This workbook will help you start to incorporate these strategies into your routine and give you a specific, individualized plan that you can use to build lifelong healthy sleep habits. Let's get started.

THE

SCIENCE

OF SLEEP

Zzzz Hush Zzzz Sleepy?
Sleep... Sleepy?

NAP Sleep... Sleepy?

DREAM * NAP DREAM

...ep... Zzz Sleep...

DREAM NAP DREAM

Zzzz Hush Zzzz
Sleepy?

Sleep... NAP Sleep... Sleepy?

DREAM * NAP DREAM

...ep... Zzz Sleep...

DREAM NAP DREAM

CHAPTER 1

INSOMNIA, BRIEFLY

IN THIS CHAPTER, I will define insomnia and its subtypes. I will also identify and describe common reasons why we may be unable to sleep. We'll discuss why sleep is important, the typical structure of sleep, the functions of various sleep phases, and the many benefits of deep, restorative sleep. I will also explain the many benefits of adequate sleep, as well as the many risks associated with lack of sleep or poor-quality sleep. Finally, you'll discover how this book and program will help you develop better sleeping habits. Let's get started on learning more about insomnia so we can work to reduce it.

SLEEPLESS NIGHTS

Greg has been struggling with insomnia for many months. He has a hard time falling asleep and staying asleep and has not been able to find a long-term solution. Often it feels like his natural energy stores don't line up with his life routine and obligations. He is exhausted at 2 p.m., 5 p.m., and 7 p.m., but then is wide awake when he is trying to go to bed at 10 p.m. Sometimes his mind is active until 2 a.m. Sometimes as he's drifting off, he has an "oh-no" moment—when his brain reminds him of worries that would be better ignored or at least dealt with in the light of day. And when the alarm goes off and wakes him at 7 a.m., he would pay a million dollars to stay in bed for another hour, but he must drag himself out of bed to get to work on time.

Greg knows he's not functioning as well as he used to. He feels exhausted much of the time and is often irritable. He cancels weekend and evening plans with friends and spends most evenings on the couch watching TV or in his bed because he is too tired to do anything else. He's stopped going to the gym due to lack of energy. He's finding it harder to focus at work and is making more mistakes on his assignments.

Greg's life now seems to revolve around sleep: thinking about it, worrying about whether he will get it, worrying about what is happening to him and his body without it, researching it on the Internet, and trying to find the antidote. He's tried most over-the-counter sleep aids and has read about sleep hygiene, but nothing he's tried has proven useful. Sometimes he feels like things are getting a little better, but it's easy to slip back to sleepless clock-watching. Despite his deep desire for sleep most of the time, he has come to dread bedtime because he knows he's likely to be in for another night of stress and frustration.

Part of why Greg is obsessed with his lack of sleep is because he knows what's at stake. He knows the long-term health consequences are real. He is also feeling the physical and mental effects of sleep deprivation daily. He's had deep, restorative sleep before, and he wants it back.

DEFINING INSOMNIA

We all have sleep disturbances from time to time, and while the occasional sleepless night is not fun, it's also not terribly unusual or disruptive. Insomnia is different because it is a recurring or consistent difficulty with falling asleep, staying asleep, or both. According to the *Diagnostic and Statistical Manual of Mental Disorders*, insomnia is the most common sleep disorder; one-third of adults report insomnia symptoms. In onset insomnia (also known as initial insomnia), individuals are not able to fall asleep quickly and may spend long periods of time trying to get to sleep. In maintenance insomnia, individuals wake much earlier than desired and have difficulty getting back to sleep. Often people have a combination of both onset and maintenance insomnia, as well as fitful sleep (tossing and turning throughout the night). Nonrestorative sleep, or poor sleep quality, leaves an individual feeling unrested and fatigued despite adequate time in bed. This is a common complaint for those who suffer from insomnia. Insomnia can be very impactful: It contributes to daytime sleepiness and fatigue and affects our mood, cognitive functioning, physical functioning, longevity, and quality of life.

The primary types of insomnia include:

ACUTE: Acute insomnia lasts only for a few days or weeks and is most often the direct result of sleep schedule changes or stressful life events. Most people will encounter acute insomnia at some point in their lives.

EARLY: Early insomnia lasts for less than one month. Factors such as situational stress, illness, or injury, as well as environmental or schedule changes, are often responsible for early insomnia.

CHRONIC: When sleeplessness lasts for at least one month it is referred to as chronic insomnia. Left untreated, chronic insomnia can last for many months or even years. Factors such as maladaptive habits and unhelpful or alarming thoughts and attitudes are largely responsible for maintaining sleeplessness in chronic insomnia.

COMORBID: It is not unusual for insomnia to occur in combination with another medical or mental health condition. Common conditions or diagnoses that occur in conjunction with insomnia are diabetes, coronary heart disease, chronic pain, anxiety, depression, and substance use disorders. In many cases, the comorbid condition is a primary cause of insomnia.

COMMON CAUSES OF INSOMNIA

There are many reasons why we may be unable to get good sleep. Often, many factors combine to cause and maintain insomnia. Here are some common causes of insomnia:

Low Sleep Drive: The physiological sleep drive is the body's craving or pressure for sleep. Our sleep drive is lowered as we sleep, and it increases with each hour we are awake. So, napping and sleeping in on the weekends, for example, can lower sleep drive in problematic ways.

Circadian Rhythm Issues: All animals have internal biological clocks that regulate multiple physiological processes. The primary clock in humans is located in the brain, and it receives information about the environment as light enters our eyes. This internal clock regulates our circadian rhythms, which adhere to a roughly 24-hour cycle. These rhythms influence periods of drowsiness and alertness throughout the day and night—for example, when the sun goes down and we are exposed to darkness, melatonin (a hormone that makes us sleepy) is released in the brain, promoting sleep. When we are exposed to light, melatonin release is suppressed. Cortisol, a stress hormone, is typically released in the early morning, bringing with it wakefulness. In addition, decreases in core body temperature that happen when it gets dark help us fall asleep and stay asleep. Situational factors such as shift work, schedule changes, stress, and temperature can disrupt or cause misalignment among our internal rhythms.

Depression: In their book *The Insomnia Answer*, insomnia treatment experts Dr. Paul Glovinsky and Dr. Arthur Spielman explain that sleep disturbance is a common symptom of depression, and depression is linked with changes in sleep architecture, or structure, that often include a phase advance in REM sleep (when REM occurs earlier than normal in the cycle). When this phase advance happens, a person's sleep span shortens to four to five hours. Sleep disturbance in depression typically includes either hypersomnia (wanting to sleep all the time) or insomnia (wakefulness in the middle of the night or early in the morning). Depression can cause sleep disturbance, and sleep problems can cause or contribute to depressive symptoms.

Anxiety and Worry: Anxiety is an emotion or feeling of fear, apprehension, uneasiness, or being on edge. It can include both physiological hyperarousal (feelings of agitation, muscle tension, and racing heart) and cognitive hyperarousal (future-oriented worries such as thinking about tomorrow's to-do list, imagining bad things that could happen, or obsessive thinking or racing thoughts). Sleep is a state of relative stillness and reduced arousal while anxiety is a state of activation and vigilance, and an anxious mind and body has difficulty finding sleep.

Unhelpful Thoughts, Beliefs, and Attitudes about Sleep: When someone has been experiencing an extended period of sleeplessness, worries about sleep and other unhelpful attitudes and beliefs can develop. This is understandable, but worrying about whether you will be able to sleep or what tomorrow will be like if you don't tends to push sleep further away.

Pain: Pain can contribute to difficulty finding a comfortable sleep position. People with chronic medical conditions often wake up due to pain or discomfort. Pain is a stressor and may cause tension and anxiety, making sleep more difficult. It is not uncommon for a vicious cycle to develop, where pain and physical discomfort lead to a lack of restorative sleep, which then increases pain and lowers physical activity and exercise, which contributes to more pain and more insomnia, and so on.

Nighttime Routine: It is not unusual for people to engage in activities that make it difficult for sleep to happen. The blue light from screens can inhibit melatonin release and make it difficult to fall asleep. Exercising and eating late can also be problematic.

Sleep Environment: Many times our sleep environment does not support deep, restorative sleep. Noise from the street, neighbors, or a partner can keep us awake. Other common causes include an uncomfortable bed, temperature issues, or a lack of darkness due to light from screens or other sources.

Substances: Caffeine, nicotine, sugar, alcohol, medications, and recreational drugs can impact our sleep in a variety of ways. Caffeine, nicotine, and sugar are stimulants, and having them late in the day can make it difficult to fall asleep and stay asleep. Alcohol may make it easier to fall asleep, but it disrupts the natural sleep cycle and can cause poor sleep quality, in part by keeping us from entering the deepest, most restorative phase of sleep.

Why do you think (or know) you can't sleep?

CONSULT YOUR PHYSICIAN

Attention! What looks and feels like insomnia could be another sleep condition such as sleep apnea, restless legs syndrome, or many others. Additionally, insomnia can be the result of other medical conditions such as diabetes, neurological conditions, or a chronic pain condition that need to be addressed. Chronic insomnia can also impact our health and contribute to the development of medical conditions. If you have been experiencing chronic, long-term insomnia, or are having emotional or physical issues because of sleeplessness, or suspect you may have another sleep disorder, it is important to discuss these issues with your physician. Ultimately, you may need to see a sleep medicine physician and have an overnight sleep study (polysomnography) to diagnose or rule out another sleep condition.

OTHER CONDITIONS THAT MAY IMPACT SLEEP

Mental Health Conditions

There are many factors that contribute to insomnia. Here is more information on a range of mental health conditions that can impact sleep as well as other sleep disorders. Many strategies in this book can help you better manage or reduce anxiety and depression and their negative impacts on sleep. However, if you think you have one of the mental health conditions below, it's important to seek evaluation and treatment from a trained mental health provider. CBT has been shown to be very effective for these conditions. In some cases, medication also greatly improves symptoms.

GENERALIZED ANXIETY DISORDER (GAD): Also known as the worry disorder and is characterized by excessive, uncontrollable worry and anxiety about a number of events or situations.

POST-TRAUMATIC STRESS DISORDER (PTSD): Characterized by exposure to a traumatic event and subsequent symptoms including distressing memories or dreams about the event, distress or physiological reactions to reminders of the event, avoidance of reminders, changes in mood and cognition, and increased physiological arousal.

MAJOR DEPRESSIVE DISORDER (MDD): Characterized by periods of low mood or sadness and/or loss of interest in pleasant activities. Other symptoms include fatigue, sleep changes, appetite or weight changes, feelings of worthlessness or guilt, difficulty thinking or concentrating, change in activity, and recurrent thoughts of death or suicide.

BIPOLAR DISORDERS: Characterized by periods of depressive symptoms and periods of mania or hypomania. Manic symptoms include elevated mood or irritability, decreased sleep, increased self-esteem, talkativeness, racing thoughts, distractibility, increased goal-directed behavior, impulsivity, and risky behavior.

OBSESSIVE-COMPULSIVE DISORDER (OCD): Characterized by the presence of *obsessions* (persistent thoughts, urges, or impulses that are intrusive and cause distress) and/or *compulsions* (repetitive behaviors or mental acts that the individual performs to reduce distress).

Other Sleep Disorders

Insomnia is the most common sleep disorder, but over 100 other sleep disorders exist and sometimes what looks like insomnia is actually something else. Below are brief descriptions of some other common sleep disorders. If you think you may have one of the disorders below, it is strongly recommended that you see a board-certified sleep physician for assessment and treatment.

SLEEP APNEA: Characterized by repeated long pauses in breathing. Untreated, it can lead to serious medical issues. Signs of sleep apnea include frequent, loud snoring, waking up gasping for air, excessive daytime sleepiness, waking up with a headache, and waking up with a dry mouth (due to sleeping with your mouth open).

RESTLESS LEGS SYNDROME (RLS): Characterized by an irresistible urge to move your legs because of an uncomfortable, odd, or crawling sensation that typically occurs in the evening while lying down.

PERIODIC LIMB MOVEMENT DISORDER: Characterized by repetitive involuntary limb movements, mostly in the lower extremities, that disrupt sleep. The movements are often brief muscle twitches, flexing, or jerking movements that the individual is not aware of.

SLEEPINESS VERSUS FATIGUE

Sleepiness is the feeling that you could fall asleep. The feeling typically increases the longer we stay awake but can be impacted by factors other than amount of time we are awake. Sleepiness is different from fatigue or exhaustion, and it's possible to feel very fatigued but not sleepy. Often people with insomnia *want* to feel sleepy at bedtime but don't. Fatigue, on the other hand, is characterized by low energy and a diminished ability for work or exertion and a need for rest but not necessarily sleep. It's important to distinguish between sleepiness and fatigue. Excessive daytime sleepiness is a common complaint with insomnia, and it is natural to feel sleepy if your sleep at night is not restorative. However, excessive daytime sleepiness can also be a sign of another sleep disorder such as sleep apnea, restless legs syndrome, or periodic limb movement disorder.

WHY WE NEED SLEEP

There is much we do not know about sleep, but innovative research is contributing to a growing knowledge about how sleep works and why we need it. Typical sleep structure, also known as sleep architecture, contains both rapid eye movement (REM) and non-rapid eye movement (NREM) stages that we cycle through about every 90 minutes. In most adults, good quality sleep tends to involve four to six of these 90-minute cycles.

The stages of sleep are qualitatively different from each other and provide our minds and bodies with different things. The deepest, most restorative sleep happens in the later NREM stages, known as slow-wave deep sleep. These deeper stages seem to be the most crucial stage of sleep and are a period of profound rest and recovery for our bodies and minds. When someone in a sleep-deprived state finally falls asleep, their brain will attempt to recover or recoup the deeper stages of sleep first. During this deep sleep our brains are relatively inactive, but important things seem to be happening in the body, such as muscle tissue repair and replenishing of energy.

After deep sleep, we enter REM sleep, where dreaming happens. REM sleep may help us process information and consolidate memories. A preponderance of research shows us that sleep helps us stay healthy and supports mental and physical well-being. Immune functioning is regulated by sleep, our need for sleep increases when we are ill, and without enough solid sleep, we are more susceptible to becoming ill.

Additionally, the risks of little or poor-quality sleep go beyond catching a common cold. A large amount of research, including many review articles and meta-analyses (examinations of data from multiple independent studies to identify overall trends) suggests that a lack of restorative sleep, over time, is associated with a greater risk of death and many other adverse health outcomes, including cancer, diabetes, cardiovascular disease, hypertension, obesity, chronic pain, cognitive decline, and respiratory disorders.

In his book *Why We Sleep*, neuroscientist and sleep researcher Matthew Walker calls sleep *the* universal health care provider, protecting us from cancer, dementia, and a host of other ailments. Without adequate restorative sleep, we are also more likely to experience anxiety and irritability and have more difficulty regulating our emotions.

Sleep deprivation is also associated with poorer concentration and increased cognitive errors and reduced motor functioning. In fact, the findings of behavioral health and safety researchers Ann Williamson and Anne-Marie Feyer, published in *Occupational and Environmental Medicine*, suggest that sleep deprivation causes impairments in cognitive and motor functioning that are equivalent to those seen in individuals with blood alcohol levels above the legal levels of intoxication, and drowsy driving is a far-too-common cause of fatal car accidents. Even more disturbing, a study conducted by a team of researchers from the University of Pennsylvania School of Medicine and Harvard Medical School and published in the journal *Sleep* found that we tend to not recognize that we are impaired when we are sleep deprived.

HOW THIS BOOK CAN HELP

Remember our friend Greg from the beginning of the chapter? He has been suffering from chronic insomnia and wants help. This book was created for Greg and the millions of other people who suffer from insomnia like you. No matter what level of insomnia you are experiencing, I'm hoping that this book will help you. The main objectives of this book are to:

- Help you identify your specific sleep issues, patterns, and problematic behaviors by looking at your sleep assessment and sleep logs.
- Teach you specific skills, coping strategies, and techniques that support restorative sleep.
- Help you reduce unhelpful behaviors, change your thinking, and build new habits.
- Maintain a process approach where we build on what is learned and view both successes and failures as necessary parts of the learning process.
- Identify and find solutions to barriers.
- Address underlying issues contributing to poor-quality sleep.
- Help you create your own individualized sleep plan.

In the final week of the program, you can reflect on what has been useful and you will be guided through the creation of a long-term sleep plan that's specific to your individual needs. We will discuss ways to maintain gains and continue to implement learned skills and strategies so that they become long-term lifestyle habits. I want to help you create these long-term habits and reap all the benefits of solid, healthy, life-enhancing sleep.

MOVING FORWARD

This chapter focused on the many benefits of adequate, restorative sleep and the consequences and long-term risks associated with a lack of good-quality sleep. We've defined insomnia and its subtypes. We've reviewed some of the most common causes of insomnia and why these factors have negative impacts on sleep. We've discussed why we need deep, restorative sleep and outlined how this book can help you build a wide range of healthy sleep habits. The next chapter will provide an introduction and overview of the main components of the four-week program.

How are you feeling about getting started?

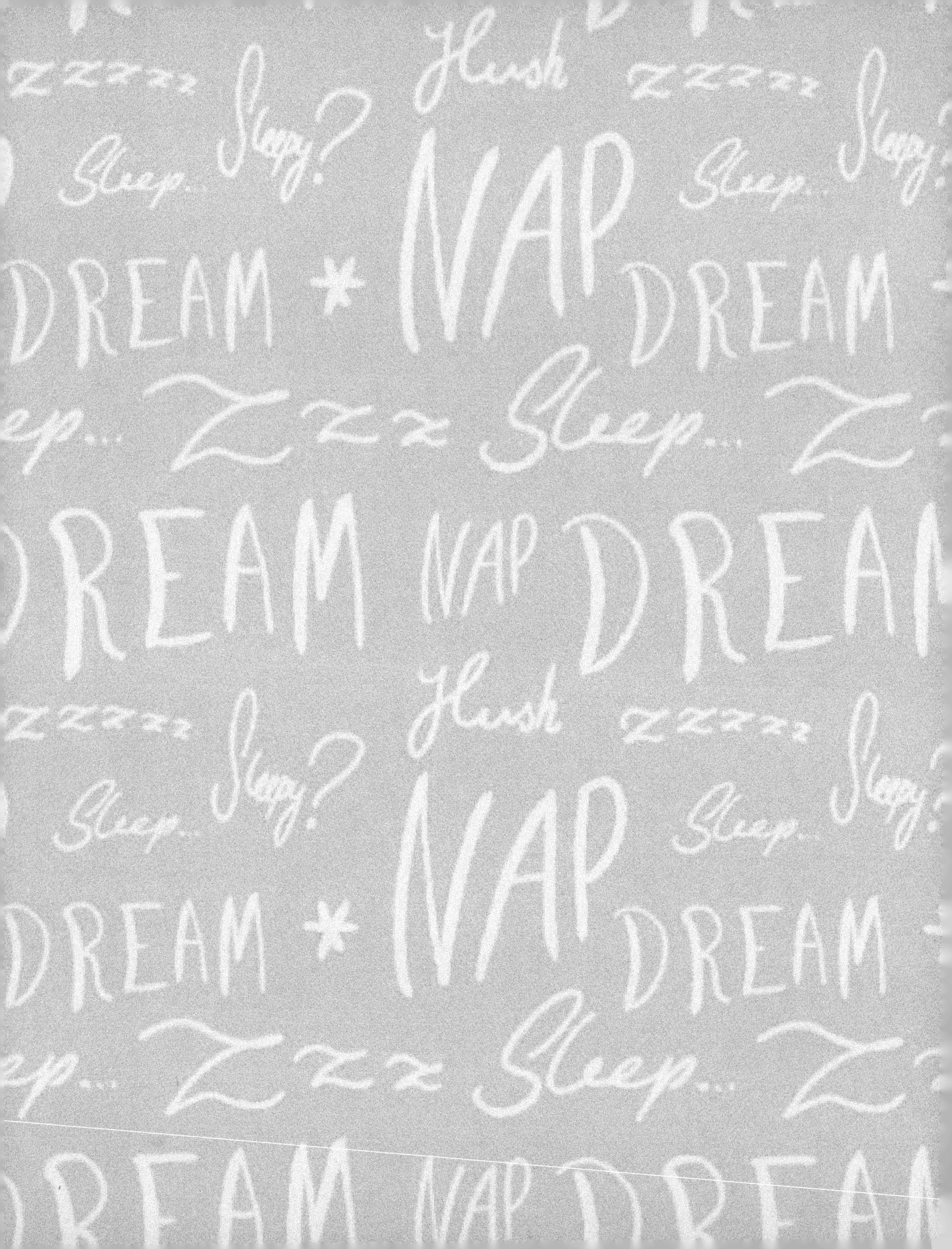
Zzzzz
Hush
Sleepy?
Sleep...
NAP
DREAM
Zzz
Sleep...

CHAPTER 2

SLEEP TECHNIQUES

THIS CHAPTER PROVIDES AN OVERVIEW of the various interventions this program has to offer. These interventions are backed by scientific research and have been shown to be effective for improving both the quantity and quality of sleep. In the following pages, we will discuss cognitive-behavioral sleep strategies, mindfulness and acceptance, relaxation, and other complementary tools. The goal here is to be both comprehensive and concise—we will dig into the specifics of how and when to apply these tools in part 2 of the workbook.

SLEEPLESS NIGHTS

Maria has been struggling with insomnia "off and on for years." She is exhausted, mildly depressed, and concerned about what years of poor sleep has done to her body and mind. Maria is feeling hopeless that things can get better. Sometimes she can string together two or three nights of decent sleep in a row—often while traveling for work or vacation—but it has never lasted. Most nights she falls asleep easily but wakes up once or twice between 12 a.m. and 3 a.m. for at least an hour or two before returning to fitful, fragmented sleep until her alarm brutally sounds at 6:30 a.m. She has tried everything. Medications and herbal supplements have not given her relief. She was already using earplugs and a fan
for white noise and temperature control. She exercises daily and drinks alcohol sparingly. She knows that looking at her phone in the middle of the night is bad for sleep but finds it hard to resist the relief it offers after tossing and turning for an hour or more. She knows that caffeine intake and naps are contributing to the cycle of insomnia but doesn't know another way to survive. Her nighttime brain is skilled at reminding her of problems at work, her list of to-dos, and worries about bad things that could happen tomorrow, the next day, or far into the future. She tries to clear her mind and stop herself from worrying, but the problems always seem bigger and brighter at 3 a.m. After the recent months of suffering, Maria had reached her limit.

CBT-I

Cognitive behavioral therapy (CBT) is a form of psychological treatment that has been around for several decades and has been applied to many types of problems that humans experience. The two earliest forms of CBT were developed in the 1950s and '60s by two American psychotherapists, Dr. Aaron Beck and Dr. Albert Ellis. Ellis believed that human suffering is not due to unfortunate circumstances or events but rather to the unhelpful ways in which people interpret and respond to these events. He thought that distorted or self-defeating beliefs are of primary importance. Similarly, Beck theorized that our automatic thoughts about ourselves, the world, and the future strongly influence our emotional states and behaviors.

Today, CBT is an umbrella term for many different types of therapies focused on the relationship between thoughts (cognition), feelings (emotion), and actions (behavior). These therapies are diverse and work in a variety of ways. Some types of CBT are focused on helping people identify and change negative or maladaptive thinking, which in turn changes feelings and problem behaviors. Other types of CBT place less emphasis on changing the content of thoughts and are more interested in changing our relationship with our thoughts. It often includes skill building, problem-solving, and home practice. A huge body of research has shown that CBT is effective for many types of mental health and physical issues, such as depression, anxiety, anger, chronic pain, drug and alcohol abuse, and eating disorders (to name just a few).

CBT for insomnia (or CBT-I) applies the main principles of CBT to the problem of insomnia by targeting the specific beliefs and behaviors that keep individuals from solid, restorative sleep. The cognitive component of CBT-I helps people notice, change, or cope better with the thoughts, worries, and beliefs that make it harder to sleep. The behavioral components of CBT-I help people develop behavioral strategies, skills, and habits that make it easier to sleep. Due to the ample research supporting its effectiveness, CBT-I has become a first line of defense against insomnia. Below are four main components of the treatment.

ADDRESSING THOUGHTS AND BEHAVIORS: CBT-I can help you identify, challenge, and work skillfully with thoughts and beliefs that may be contributing to your insomnia. It also targets the specific behaviors that make it difficult to get deep, uninterrupted sleep.

STIMULUS CONTROL: After a long period of insomnia, our brains and bodies may have learned to be awake during the times that we want and need to be asleep. Stimulus control training is a behaviorally-based component of CBT-I that retrains your brain to recognize that nighttime and your bedroom are for sleep.

SLEEP RESTRICTION: Sometimes reducing the number of hours you are in bed helps to consolidate sleep so that it is less fitful and more refreshing. As your sleep quality and efficiency improve, you will slowly increase the amount of time you spend in bed until you reach your goal.

SLEEP HYGIENE: Sleep hygiene guidelines help you create or break habits and set up your sleep environment in a way that supports reliable, restorative sleep.

Mindfulness and mindful awareness are woven into many cognitive behavioral interventions, including this treatment program. Mindfulness can also be used and has been shown to be effective as a stand-alone intervention for not only insomnia but other conditions that impact sleep, such as chronic pain and anxiety. Relaxation techniques work to calm the mind and the body and have also been shown to be useful in improving sleep. Other (external) tools that may be effective, depending on the cause of insomnia, include light therapy devices, sound machines, and smartphone apps.

Mindfulness and Meditation

Mindfulness means paying attention to the present moment in a nonjudgmental, accepting, and compassionate way. It is not goal-oriented; it is a mode of being. It is about acceptance, not achievement. Mindfulness is an awareness of what is happening without striving or grasping for change. Generally, it helps to do three things: Notice and change self-defeating patterns, accept and regulate difficult emotions and sensations, and be more aware of and less controlled by emotions, urges, and impulses. These skills have been shown to be effective for coping with and reducing insomnia.

When we are not sleeping, it is easy to become stressed about the sleep we are not getting. Stress, anxiety, worry, and frustration about sleep make sleep even more elusive. Mindfulness helps reduce stress, and part of mindful awareness is about observing and accepting what is happening while trying not to judge it (and not getting caught up in worry). Mindfulness meditation is a formal practice that helps cultivate the skills of mindful awareness. Some examples of classic formal mindfulness meditations include breath awareness, the body scan, and metta (lovingkindness or compassion) meditation. These are really useful tools that can enhance sleep hygiene and be used in combination with other cognitive behavioral interventions. See "Week 3" for instructions for the mindful breath meditation (page 77) and the body scan (pages 80 to 81). The more you practice these skills and take notice of what works for you over time, the more beneficial they'll become.

Relaxation Methods

Relaxation techniques are also very useful for improving sleep. They are a bit different from meditation or mindfulness strategies in that they are much more goal-oriented. The goal is to relax the body and mind, to let go of and reduce tension. Relaxation methods work by turning down our body's stress response, known as the fight-or-flight response, that's driven by the sympathetic nervous system and activating the recovery or relaxation response via the parasympathetic nervous system. Specific relaxation exercises include progressive muscle relaxation (PMR) and guided imagery or visualization. Gentle yoga practices, such as hatha yoga, may also be useful in activating the relaxation response.

External Tools

External tools, such as light therapy boxes, meditation apps, or noise machines, may also be something you'll want to explore. These tools can be used in combination with cognitive behavioral interventions and may enhance treatment. The dosing and timing of light therapy is very important and varies depending on the specific sleep issue. Light therapy should also be discussed with your physician, as there may be side effects or contraindications.

EXERCISE: IMAGERY AND VISUALIZATION

You can use your imagination to work more effectively with inner experiences that may be contributing to insomnia (such as pain or anxiety). Imagery and visualization exercises can powerfully change your experience. It's helpful to pull in as many of your senses as possible (sight, smell, sound, and touch) to deepen the experience. Here is one exercise you can practice.

Visualize Your Pain

This exercise can be used to manage both physical and emotional pain or discomfort. First, locate where in your body you feel the physical or emotional pain. If it is an emotion, identify it. Now, imagine this pain has a physical form. Give it a shape and a color. Notice its size. Picture this form as clearly as you can. Now, slow the pace of your breath but continue to breathe in a way that feels comfortable and natural. Imagine that you can breathe directly into the discomfort you've visualized, and as you breathe, you are able to change its form to something more comfortable. You are bringing compassionate care to yourself as you breathe. Maybe the form is changing color. You could imagine gently moving the form to another part of your body or shrinking its size. In this visualization you can get really creative and experiment with changing the image, while continuing to breathe in a way that is comfortable and soothing.

Take a closer look at these methods. Are you familiar with any of them? Which ones do you feel drawn to or comfortable trying? Which ones feel more challenging?

_____

_____

_____

_____

ACCEPTANCE AND COMMITMENT THERAPY

Acceptance and commitment therapy (often pronounced "act" in the psychology world) is a cognitive behavioral treatment based on scientific research about how the human mind works. The name of this therapy comes from a primary theme: learning how to accept those experiences that are out of your control and committing to changing what you can to make your life better. The basic principles are very helpful when applied to insomnia. Acceptance of sleeplessness is extremely useful. In ACT, we talk about stopping the battle with sleeplessness because the battle itself can be maddening, and it adds an extra layer of suffering on top of the sleeplessness. Chasing sleep doesn't tend to work. We don't capture sleep; we surrender to it. Acceptance of what is happening in the moment is part of the process of working skillfully with insomnia. In ACT, you don't fight with insomnia. You work with it. This includes making some changes to how you behave and how you relate to your thoughts and feelings about being awake when you would rather be asleep. Sometimes making these changes is difficult. This is where values and commitment come in. Ask yourself: Why do you want to make changes to get better sleep? Is it about being healthy? Being more present at work or in your relationships? Having more energy so that you can do more things that bring you satisfaction, meaning, or a sense of vitality? Clarifying *why* making these changes is important to *you* and highlighting that for yourself can help you commit to taking action and sticking with it.

SLEEP AIDS*

This book takes a drug-free approach to helping you get better quality sleep. However, it's understood that in some cases medications or supplements may be useful or necessary. While we cannot recommend sleep aids—anything you take should be either prescribed or recommended by your personal physician—here are a few that are commonly used. Make sure you have a full understanding of how these may interact with any other medication or supplement you take and how they may affect you overall. This is not an exhaustive list, nor is it medical advice. All of these aids have some risks of side effects and may not be recommended for children, adolescents, or individuals with certain medical conditions, or who are pregnant or breast-feeding. Additionally, "natural" herbs and supplements may seem safer but are often unregulated and not well-researched. Please use this section as a way to start a conversation with your physician about your options.

Prescriptions

TRAZODONE: An antidepressant medication that is also regularly prescribed for sleep. It acts by impacting serotonin and its receptors and is considered safe for longer-term use and is not considered habit-forming. Notable side effects include GI symptoms (such as nausea and vomiting), sedation, edema, blurred vision, dry mouth, constipation, dizziness, fatigue, headache, incoordination, tremor, cardiovascular changes, and, rarely, rash.

ZOLPIDEM (AMBIEN): A sedative-hypnotic sleep medication that is commonly prescribed for the short-term treatment of insomnia. It generally takes effect in less than an hour. When it works, it tends to reduce nighttime awakening and the time it takes to fall asleep. Notable side effects include sedation, dizziness, dose-dependent amnesia, and nervousness and hyperexcitability. Rare side effects include (but are not limited to) hallucinations, GI symptoms (such as nausea), and headache. There is a risk of becoming dependent on the drug over time.

ESZOPICLONE (LUNESTA): Another sedative-hypnotic sleep medication that is commonly prescribed for acute and chronic insomnia. Like Ambien, it generally takes effect in less than an hour, and when effective, there is a decrease in the time it takes to fall asleep and nighttime awakenings. Notable side effects include (but are not limited to)

* Adapted from *Essential Psychopharmacology Prescriber's Guide*, 6th Ed., by Stephen M. Stahl. See also the National Sleep Foundation website (https://www.sleepfoundation.org).

unpleasant taste, sedation, dose-dependent amnesia, nervousness, dry mouth, and headache. Life-threatening side effects include respiratory depression, especially when taken with other central nervous system depressants, and, rarely, angioedema. There is a risk of becoming dependent on the drug over time.

SUVOREXANT (BELSOMRA): A new sleep medication that targets a different chemical in the brain. It is an orexin receptor antagonist, which means that it works by blocking the effects of the chemical orexin, which promotes alertness and wakefulness. It generally takes effect within one hour, and theoretically works by improving quality of sleep and reducing wakefulness and nighttime awakenings. Notable side effects include sedation, headaches, dizziness, and abnormal dreams. Rare but dangerous or life-threatening side effects include sleep paralysis and hallucinations and symptoms similar to cataplexy.

CLONAZEPAM (KLONOPIN) AND LORAZEPAM (ATIVAN): Both are benzodiazepine medications most commonly prescribed for anxiety and seizure disorders but also commonly prescribed for sleep. They tend to work very quickly for anxiety and are considered habit-forming. Notable side effects include (but are not limited to) depression, dizziness, ataxia, slurred speech, weakness, forgetfulness, confusion, excitability, nervousness, and, rarely, hallucinations, mania, hypotension, and hypersalivation or dry mouth.

Over-the-Counter

DIPHENHYDRAMINE OR DPH (E.G., BENADRYL, ALEVE PM, ZZZQUIL): This is an antihistamine. You probably think of allergies and immune system reactions when you think about taking an antihistamine. Antihistamines work by blocking histamine, which is a neurotransmitter that not only impacts immune reactions but also the sleep-wake cycle. Histamine promotes arousal and alertness, and the antihistamine diphenhydramine is sedating. Some possible side effects include morning hangover, dry mouth, urinary retention, constipation, and blurred vision.

DOXYLAMINE SUCCINATE (UNISOM): Another sedating antihistamine with side effects similar to diphenhydramine.

Herbals and Supplements

MELATONIN: A hormone primarily produced in the brain that is released when the sun goes down. Our levels of melatonin typically stay high throughout the night and are low during the day. There is wide dispute about the effectiveness of synthetic melatonin for insomnia. It may be more effective for jet lag and disrupted sleep due to shift work. Side effects include headache and daytime sleepiness.

VALERIAN: A tall flowering plant, and its root is a popular herbal supplement for insomnia, as well as anxiety, pain relief, and various other issues. There is disagreement regarding valerian's effectiveness for the treatment of insomnia. Evidence from a meta-analysis of 16 research studies (Bent et al. 2015) suggests that valerian may improve sleep quality without side effects. However, most of those studies have significant methodological problems or limitations. Other evidence indicates that valerian's side effects include headache, morning hangover, upset stomach, restlessness, and irregular heartbeat. Additionally, valerian may interact with many other medications and substances, and using valerian in combination with other sedating substances, including alcohol, can be quite dangerous. Individuals with liver problems may be advised to avoid valerian.

CANNABIDIOL (CBD): A nonintoxicating cannabis extract. It is taken from marijuana and hemp plants but does not give you the "high" of marijuana, because it does not contain the psychoactive chemical THC. CBD is becoming quickly popular for many ailments, including epilepsy, chronic pain, and anxiety, and it is widely available, but its exact legal status is in flux and varies from state to state. When it works, CBD may help people fall asleep more quickly and stay asleep. Anecdotal reports suggest that CBD may be more effective for insomnia if you take it right before you turn the lights out and go to bed. As with other herbs and supplements, the research on CBD is quite limited, it is not FDA regulated, and the quality of the product can vary widely. It is important to be cautious of interaction effects, as there is evidence that CBD has an inhibiting effect on other pharmaceuticals. In other words, CBD can reduce the effectiveness of other medications. It may also increase levels of some medications (like blood thinners) in your blood. Noted side effects include nausea, fatigue, and irritability.

CHAMOMILE TEA: A naturally caffeine-free tea and known anecdotally for its relaxing effects. It's been used for centuries for a variety of issues, including sleep and anxiety. The scientific data supporting chamomile's effectiveness for insomnia is limited. However, many people swear by it, and the ritual of making a cup of tea and drinking something warm can be a relaxing practice. Some side effects of chamomile include nausea, vomiting, allergic reaction, and blood thinner interference.

Sleep aids often help us fall asleep, but many over-the-counter and prescription sleep aids inhibit our bodies from entering the deepest stages of sleep or getting enough REM sleep. Some sleep aids mask our natural sleep tendencies or produce hangovers the next day. Additionally, if you take a sleep aid nightly and suddenly stop, you may experience "rebound insomnia," a transient period of increased arousal and disrupted sleep. Sometimes the rebound insomnia causes people to experience far worse sleep than before they started taking the sleep aid, which contributes to the perception that they cannot sleep without the help of a sleep aid.

If you are taking a sleep aid, or are considering using one, it is important that you have a full understanding of how they work. Please discuss this with your physician if you want to learn more. The goal of this book is to help you establish new habits that promote restorative sleep.

What are your experiences with sleep aids and your current thoughts and concerns about sleep aids?

GETTING COMFORTABLE WITH DISCOMFORT

If you are feeling a bit overwhelmed by the prospect of taking on your insomnia, I get it. We are going to take on the challenge of insomnia together. It may require making some significant changes and breaking longtime habits. Participation in this program may involve noticing thoughts and feelings that are painful. You may need to give up some immediate comforts and experience short-term discomfort for the sake of achieving longer-term, lasting rewards. Participation takes some real effort and requires some tracking and recordkeeping of daily habits and sleep patterns. Making these kinds of changes requires a certain amount of patience and willingness to be uncomfortable and a strong commitment to the process. But I think full participation, putting forth your best effort, is worth it. I have seen how CBT-I can make a big impact on someone's ability to sleep and their overall quality of life.

Are you ready to commit? If you are feeling unsure, I understand. Uncertainty or ambivalence is a normal and often necessary part of this process. It is essential that you are compassionate with yourself as you contemplate taking steps to make your life better. Here are things to consider that may encourage you to commit to the program.

Consider Your Rewards

Deciding to make changes and fully engaging in this program can be a great act of self-care and self-kindness. It will not happen overnight, but CBT-I has been shown to be effective in reducing insomnia and you have a good chance of success if you stick to the program. There is no guarantee that any treatment will work the way we hope it will, but research shows us that there is good reason to be optimistic that CBT-I will work for you.

Understanding That There's No One "Right" Way to Sleep

This is not a one-size-fits-all program. We are giving you the best cognitive behavioral therapy has to offer for eliminating insomnia, but we understand that everyone has their own unique sleep goals. If going to bed at 2 a.m. and waking up at 11 a.m. works for you and your schedule, do that. The strategies in this book can be adapted for your ideal lifestyle.

Go at Your Own Pace

Again, flexibility is very useful when participating in this program. If the four-week structure outlined here doesn't work for you, take your time with the material. You might start with an aspect of sleep hygiene that you feel the most willing to take on. Start with what feels right. This is not a race or a competition. And perfection is not the goal. The goal is to build habits that will lead to lifestyle changes. It may take a bit longer for some of us. It's not unusual to have setbacks and false starts. That is okay! It is essential to view change as a process. I want you to see failures and false starts as an important part of this process, loaded with valuable information. Take that new information you gained from any failures and try again.

Are you ready to fully commit to making changes in order to get better sleep? What might help you cope with potential challenges as they arise?

MOVING FORWARD

This chapter gave a broad overview of the various components that we will explore to help you break the pattern of insomnia. The program will offer the most effective sleep interventions CBT has to offer—interventions that are backed by research and that have been shown to improve sleep. We've introduced behavioral interventions such as stimulus control therapy, sleep restriction therapy, and sleep hygiene. We've discussed cognitive interventions, mindfulness and relaxation, and complementary therapies and tools. Hopefully this chapter has piqued your interest and inspired some hope that your sleep habits can improve. It includes a lot of information to process, and if making changes seems daunting, please remember that flexibility and self-compassion are key.

More specifics about each of the aspects of the program will be discussed later in the book. The next chapter will introduce an extremely important step in building healthy sleep habits: establishing the baseline and ongoing assessment of your sleep needs, sleep behaviors, and sleep quality.

Zzzz Sleepy? Hush Zzzz Sleep... Sleepy?
Sleep...

DREAM ✳ NAP DREAM ✳

p... Zzz Sleep... Z

DREAM NAP DREAM

Hush Zzzz Sleepy?
Sleep... Sleepy?
Sleep...

NAP

DREAM ✳ NAP DREAM

p... Zzz Sleep... Z

DREAM NAP DREAM

CHAPTER 3

BASELINE AND SLEEP ASSESSMENT

THE PURPOSE OF THIS CHAPTER is to guide you through a self-assessment that will provide an in-depth view of your current sleep habits and detect the specific factors negatively impacting your sleep. The assessment process also involves completing brief sleep logs daily to obtain some baseline data. You will be asked to continue completing these logs daily as part of the program to reveal patterns and track your progress. At the end of the chapter we will use data from the assessment and baseline sleep logs to help you identify your specific sleep goals.

HOW MUCH SLEEP DO YOU NEED?

There is quite a bit of variation in how much people sleep and how much sleep someone needs to feel rested and energized, but we do have some information about what is average. On average, adults tend to sleep somewhere between six and eight hours at night. It typically takes people 10 to 20 minutes to fall asleep. It's normal to wake up two to three times during the night, and it often takes up to 15 minutes to fall back to sleep.

The World Health Organization recommends that adults strive to achieve eight hours of sleep each night, but the data suggests that some people need significantly more or less than this amount. We also know that teenagers need more than eight hours of sleep nightly, and older adults are typically unable to get a solid eight hours of sleep. It is important to note that just because you may be able to get by on very little sleep does not necessarily mean that you are well rested or that a lack of sleep is not impacting you. Sometimes the impact of insufficient sleep is not obvious or is being partially masked by substances like caffeine. It's very helpful to pause and take a closer look at your sleep habits and how they are working for you. As part of this, it's useful to look at factors that may be impacting both your physiological sleep drive and circadian rhythm.

EXERCISE: DETERMINING YOUR IDEAL AMOUNT OF SLEEP

Think of the last time you slept, awoke refreshed, and had plenty of energy throughout the day—or the last time in your life you were consistently getting enough solid sleep. How many hours did you sleep? What were your sleep conditions? What did your life look like? Now, take a moment to consider: If all your sleep problems were suddenly solved, how many hours of sleep would you hope to get each night? You can write your answers to these questions below:

_____

_____

_____

THE SLEEP SELF-ASSESSMENT AND SLEEP LOG

Completing "The Sleep Self-Assessment" (pages 32 to 34) and the "Daily Sleep Log" (page 36) are important first steps in building healthy sleep habits. We are going to uncover the nitty-gritty of your sleep. I want to give you a sense of what your current sleep looks like, including sleep quality, quantity, timing, patterns, and habits. This assessment will highlight potential problem areas and help you create goals and your own individualized treatment plan.

THE SLEEP LOG

The sleep log is a critical part of the baseline sleep assessment and an ongoing measure of progress toward your sleep goals and what is working.

Ideally, you will complete this log for seven days before starting the program to give you some data and help identify patterns. Fill out the log tonight before bed and when you wake up tomorrow. Again, the data from this log and the sleep assessment will help you make treatment choices and set goals tailored to your individual needs and priorities. You will be asked to complete the sleep log each evening and morning throughout the program to monitor your progress, identify barriers or problems, and assist in troubleshooting. You can find extra copies of the Daily Sleep Log in the Blank Worksheets and Forms section (see page 110) or online at www.CallistoMediaBooks.com/InsomniaWorkbook.

Instructions

This sleep log includes two sections. The top section includes some behaviors that may affect sleep and is to be completed at night, right before bed. The bottom section focuses on the timing, quality, and duration of sleep and time in bed and is to be completed each morning when you wake up.

If your schedule requires you to sleep during the day and be awake at night, complete the log at a time that lines up with your schedule. It is okay to estimate things like the time you fell asleep and how much time you spent awake. A good estimate is good enough.

There are a few calculations to be done each morning as well:

SLEEP ONSET LATENCY: The time from lights out until the time you fell asleep.

ESTIMATED TIME ASLEEP (TA): Calculated by adding up the hours from the time you fell asleep to the time you finally woke up and subtracting the time for each awakening.

THE SLEEP SELF-ASSESSMENT

INSTRUCTIONS: Please consider what your sleep and sleep habits have been like *for the past month.*

PART 1: SLEEP DURATION, EFFICIENCY, AND TIMING

During the last month:

1. On average, how many hours of sleep did you get each night? _____
2. a. On average, for how many hours were you in bed each night, both awake and asleep? _____
   b. Sleep Efficiency (Time Asleep ÷ Time in Bed) × 100 = _____%
3. On average, how long did it take you to fall asleep (Sleep Onset Latency)? _____
4. What time did you typically go to bed? _____
5. What time did you typically get up in the morning? _____

PART 2: SLEEP SYMPTOMS

Use the following scale for the questions below:

0 Never
1 Less than once a week
2 Once a week
3 2 to 3 times a week
4 4 or more times a week

During the past month, how often have you:

1. Had difficulty falling asleep? _____
2. Had difficulty staying asleep? _____
3. Woke up earlier than you wanted and weren't able to fall back to sleep quickly? _____
4. Felt your sleep quality was poor? _____
5. Felt fatigued during the day? _____
6. Canceled activities due to fatigue? _____
7. Had trouble staying awake during tasks like driving, eating, or socializing? _____

8. Relied on caffeine or other stimulants to get through the day? _____
9. Used a medication or substance to try and fall asleep? _____
   Please list what you took: _____
10. Worried about lack of sleep or not being able to sleep? _____
11. Thought about how difficult the next day would be due to lack of sleep? _____
12. Felt that an overactive mind was keeping you awake? _____
13. Felt too anxious, keyed up, or agitated to sleep? _____
14. Felt frustrated by not being able to sleep? _____
15. Had physical pain or discomfort that impacted your sleep? _____

Sleep Hygiene Factors

1. Had caffeine within 8 to 10 hours of bedtime? _____
2. Had alcohol within 3 hours of bedtime? _____
3. Napped? _____
4. Used screens while in bed (TV, phones, tablets, etc.)? _____
5. Watched TV or used other screens within one hour of bedtime? _____
6. Worked or engaged in other activities besides sleep or sex while in bed? _____
7. Felt your bedroom was too hot or cold, too noisy, or otherwise uncomfortable? _____
8. Felt that your sleep was disrupted by others (bedpartner, children, pets)? _____

Physical and Emotional Factors

1. Rate your stress level over the last month.
   (0 = no stress and 10 = extreme stress): _____
2. Rate your level of anxiety over the last month.
   (0 = no anxiety and 10 = extreme anxiety): _____
3. Rate your level of depression over the last month.
   (0 = no depression and 10 = extreme depression): _____
4. Rate your pain level over the last month.
   (0 = no pain and 10 = extreme pain): _____

Reflection Questions

1. Do you think of yourself as a morning person, an evening person, or somewhere in between?

2. How well does your natural sleep schedule or timing preference align with your life obligations? For example, what if you would prefer to stay up late and sleep late, but your family, work, school, or social obligations require you get up early? If this leads to sleep deprivation, there could be poor alignment.

3. How consistent is your sleep schedule? (Check one.)
   - O Very consistent
   - O Somewhat consistent
   - O Somewhat inconsistent
   - O Very inconsistent

4. What do you think impacts your sleep the most?

5. Rate the overall quality of your sleep in the past month. (Check one.)
   - O Very good
   - O Good
   - O Poor
   - O Very poor

6. Rate the impact of poor sleep on your life in the past month. (Check one.)
   - O No impact
   - O Mild
   - O Moderate
   - O Severe

DAILY SLEEP LOG EXAMPLE*

Date: _1-15-2019_

PART 1: COMPLETE IN THE EVENING, BEFORE BED

How many caffeinated beverages? ___3___

Time of last caffeine? _1 p.m._

How many alcoholic beverages? ___0___

Time of last alcohol? _____

Did you exercise? _Yes—ran 20 min, 10 a.m._

Did you nap? _Yes—1 hr, 3 p.m._

Medications/sleep aids? _melatonin_

How fatigued were you today? (0 = no fatigue to 10 = extreme fatigue) ___7___

PART 2: COMPLETE IN THE MORNING, UPON GETTING UP

What time did you get into bed? _10 p.m._

What time was lights out? _10:30 p.m._

What time did you fall asleep? _10:45 p.m._

Sleep onset latency (time from lights out until asleep): _15 min_

Number of awakenings (not including the final time you woke up): ___2___

How long for each? 1st: _1 hr_ 2nd: _45 min_ 3rd: _____ 4th: _____ 5th: _____

Time of final wake-up? _6 a.m._

What time did you get out of bed? _6:15 a.m._

Estimated total time asleep (TA)? _5.5 hrs_

Total time in bed (TIB)? _8.25 hrs_

Sleep efficiency? ([TA ÷ TIB] ×100) _(5.5 ÷ 8.25) × 100 = 66.7%_

Quality of sleep? (0 = poor to 10 = excellent) ___3___

Pain or discomfort? (0 = no pain to 10 = extreme pain) ___0___

Stress or distress level? (0 = no distress to 10 = high distress) ___7___

Any in-bed activities? (watching TV, screens, work, reading, etc.)
re-reading work notes, reading on phone

Other notes: _stressed about presentation for work_

* Adapted from "The 60-Second Sleep Diary" in *Say Goodnight to Insomnia*, by Gregg D. Jacobs.

DAILY SLEEP LOG

Date: _____

PART 1: COMPLETE IN THE EVENING, BEFORE BED

How many caffeinated beverages? _____

Time of last caffeine? _____

How many alcoholic beverages? _____

Time of last alcohol? _____

Did you exercise? _____

Did you nap? _____

Medications/sleep aids? _____

How fatigued were you today? (0 = no fatigue to 10 = extreme fatigue) _____

PART 2: COMPLETE IN THE MORNING, UPON GETTING UP

What time did you get into bed? _____

What time was lights out? _____

What time did you fall asleep? _____

Sleep onset latency (time from lights out until asleep): _____

Number of awakenings (not including the final time you woke up): _____

How long for each? 1st: _____ 2nd: _____ 3rd: _____ 4th: _____ 5th: _____

Time of last awakening? _____

What time did you get out of bed? _____

Estimated total time asleep (TA)? _____

Total time in bed (TIB)? _____

Sleep efficiency? ([TA ÷ TIB] × 100) = _____%

Quality of sleep? (0 = poor to 10 = excellent) _____

Pain or discomfort? (0 = no pain to 10 = extreme pain) _____

Stress or Distress level? (0 = no distress to 10 = high distress) _____

Any in-bed activities? (watching TV, screens, work, reading, etc.)

_____

Other notes:

_____

TIME IN BED (TIB): The hours between the time you got into bed at night and the time you got out for the day.

SLEEP EFFICIENCY: The higher the sleep efficiency percentage, the less fragmented or interrupted your sleep. Sleep efficiency is your total hours asleep (TA) divided by your total hours in bed (TIB) multiplied by 100.

$$(TA \div TIB) \times 100 = \text{Sleep Efficiency \%}$$

SLEEP LOG SUMMARY INSTRUCTIONS*

I would also like you to complete a brief sleep log summary at the end of each week by calculating the weekly averages for sleep latency, total time in bed, total hours asleep, sleep efficiency, fatigue, stress/distress, pain/discomfort, and quality of sleep.

* Adapted from "Sleep Log Summary (Expanded)" in *End the Insomnia Struggle: A Step-by-Step Guide to Help You Get to Sleep and Stay Asleep*, by Colleen Ehrnstrom and Alisha L. Brosse.

WEEKLY SLEEP LOG SUMMARY

Week #: _____

Dates: _____

Average Sleep Onset Latency: _____

Average Estimated Time Asleep (TA): _____

Average Time in Bed (TIB): _____

Average Sleep Efficiency: ([TA ÷ TIB] × 100%) = _____%

Average number of awakenings: _____

Average fatigue: _____

Average quality of sleep: _____

Average stress/distress: _____

Average pain/discomfort: _____

SCORING THE SLEEP SELF-ASSESSMENT AND GOAL SETTING

As you look over your answers on the self-assessment, take note of items where you have a score of 3 or 4. Items with a 3 are happening with some significant consistency (at least twice a week) and items with a 4 are happening more days than not. Additionally, think about the impact of each item. For example, if you are falling asleep while driving, even infrequently, the risk and potential negative impact of this is very high. Also, using both the self-assessment and the baseline sleep log summary, take note of the average baseline amount of sleep you are getting, your sleep onset latency, the number of awakenings, fatigue level, and overall quality of sleep.

Given this data, what are your sleep goals? You want the goals to be both specific and realistic. Specificity matters because if the goal is too vague, it is difficult to know how to achieve it and whether you are making progress. Setting realistic goals reduces frustration and increases the chances that you will stick with the program and have success. Here are some goal categories to consider:

- Building healthy sleep habits to get better quality sleep and reduce fatigue. For example, you may want to increase the duration or quality of your sleep, have fewer awakenings, or increase sleep efficiency.

- Implementing cognitive and behavioral strategies and coping skills to more effectively deal with thoughts and emotions that are contributing to insomnia and reduce distress. For example, you may want to feel less stressed or anxious at night.

- Implementing cognitive and behavioral strategies and coping skills to cope better with pain or discomfort that is contributing to insomnia. For example, you may want to use relaxation to reduce muscle tension and mindfulness to battle less with physical discomfort.

Write three goals related to improving your sleep below:

Goal 1: _____

Goal 2: _____

Goal 3: _____

Is there anything surprising about your baseline results? What goal feels most important at this point?

_____

_____

_____

_____

_____

MOVING FORWARD

This chapter was all about assessment. Now you have more specific data on the quantity, quality, efficiency, and timing of your sleep, your sleep habits and behaviors, your mood and physical discomfort, and the impact of insomnia on your daily functioning. You have identified specific goals to address these issues. In the next section of the book you will begin the program by learning to build the healthy sleep habits that can improve your sleep.

Before we begin, think back to a time that was particularly challenging, or another time in your life where you needed to make a change and successfully did so. What inner resources or personal strengths helped you? How did you stay motivated?

_____

_____

_____

_____

THE

PROGRAM

Hush
Zzzzz
Sleep.. Sleepy?
NAP Sleep... Sleepy
DREAM ✳ DREAM
ep... Zzz Sleep... Z
DREAM NAP DREAM
Hush
Zzzzz
Sleep.. Sleepy?
NAP Sleep... Sleepy
DREAM ✳ DREAM
ep... Zzz Sleep... Z
DREAM NAP DREAM

CHANGING YOUR SLEEP BEHAVIORS

THIS WEEK IS ALL ABOUT LEARNING THE BASICS. We will go over a comprehensive tutorial of the behavioral components of CBT-I: good sleep hygiene, stimulus control therapy, and sleep restriction therapy. Your baseline self-assessment and sleep logs will help you decide what changes might be necessary to increase your chances of getting deep, solid, restorative sleep. You will be given the rationale for each strategy to help you think about your motivation to make changes. Many of these strategies may be familiar to you. Often, the most effective sleep interventions don't consist of one simple change like a sleeping pill, the right sound machine, or the perfect pillow. The most effective interventions are typically ones that address the whole sleep system: the mind, the body, and the environment, as well as thoughts, emotions, and behaviors. Successful interventions typically involve making a series of changes in your sleep behaviors.

NO MORE SLEEPLESS NIGHTS

Nate refers to himself as a lifelong insomniac. Now in his early forties, he cannot remember an extended period in his life when he felt well-rested and energized. His mom says that even as a baby he did not sleep well. He is likely one of those individuals with more genetic or biological vulnerabilities for insomnia. Nate thinks of himself as a night owl. However, that schedule isn't very compatible with his work and family obligations. Over the years, Nate has adopted a variety of habits to cope with sleep deprivation and the resulting fatigue. He sleeps very late on the weekends when he can, he uses caffeine to stave off midday sleepiness, and he schedules weekend activities for later in the evening, when he tends to be more alert. He would like to exercise but has not found a way to work it into his schedule. He is also fairly stressed by his job, and when he tries to go to bed early, he feels that he can't turn off his brain. He drinks alcohol to relax most evenings and finds that this does slow down his mind a bit. But he is fairly sure the alcohol is actually making his sleep worse.

Nate has read a lot about sleep hygiene and has made some changes in the past that slightly improved his sleep, but it has never lasted. However, he is ready to try again and wants to look at all of the factors that may be impacting his sleep. He wants to look at his schedule, his obligations, his sleep hygiene and habits, and his strategies for coping with both fatigue and stress. He is motivated to make changes and is ready to commit to building healthy sleep habits.

DEFINING SLEEP HYGIENE

In general, hygiene is about daily practices that keep us healthy and prevent disease. Personal hygiene includes all the basics—bathing, washing our hair, and washing our hands. In the same vein, sleep hygiene is about staying healthy by building daily practices that increase the probability that we will get good quality sleep. However, it is easy to develop habits that are enjoyable and feel restful but do not support long-term restorative sleep. This makes sense—it feels good to curl up in bed and watch a movie when you are fatigued or take a later afternoon nap when you are sleep deprived. But these types of behaviors may be perpetuating and exacerbating insomnia. In the following sections, I'll discuss some alternatives that tend to promote and support healthy sleep.

Set a Regular Sleep Schedule

Going to bed and getting up at about the same time every day, including the weekends, is a habit that will support your body's internal clock via external cues. This is discussed more in the section on stimulus control therapy (see "The Pavlov Connection: Stimulus Control Therapy," page 48). This is an important part of improving your sleep hygiene.

Reduce or Eliminate Naps

Napping during the day reduces our sleep drive, and you may want to try and give them up altogether until you reach your sleep goals. If you do need to nap, try to keep it to 20 to 30 minutes and avoid early evening naps.

Check Your Sleep Environment

It's important that you have checked the following things in your sleep environment:

- Make sure you have a comfortable bed and bedding.
- The bedroom temperature should be comfortable and cool but not cold. A common suggestion is to aim for 65 degrees Fahrenheit, which is significantly cooler than what most people are used to.
- Aim for a restful bedroom environment: quiet, dark, and free from distractions.

Monitor Substance Intake

What substances we ingest can have a huge impact on the quality and quantity of our sleep. The effects can last much longer than we realize:

CAFFEINE: works by blocking the effects of adenosine, a chemical that builds up in the body over the course of the day when we are awake. Adenosine fuels the sleep drive, and once its concentration peaks, you begin to feel very sleepy—unless, of course, caffeine is standing in the way. Caffeine has a half-life of about five to seven hours, which means that even seven hours after your last cup of coffee, you may still have up to 50 percent of that caffeine in your system. Sensitivity to caffeine and its effects varies, but if you think caffeine is a contributing factor to your insomnia, it is best to stop ingesting it as early in the day as possible—ideally before noon or even earlier. Also, remember that caffeine not only exists in coffee, soda, and some teas but also some energy drinks, medicines (including some pain relievers and decongestants), and chocolate. Decaffeinated coffee contains up to 30 percent of the caffeine in a regular cup of coffee.

NICOTINE: can cause fragmented, lighter sleep even hours after smoking. Regular smokers may also wake earlier than they want to due to nicotine withdrawal. If you smoke, quitting is one of the best things you can do for your health.

ALCOHOL: may appear to help you fall asleep, but the evidence shows us that it reduces the amount of deep sleep we experience and causes sleep to be more fitful throughout the night. Skipping the nightcap is helpful, avoiding alcohol for at least three hours before bed is even better, and for some people, not drinking alcohol at all is the best choice for sleep.

MEDICATIONS: can also impact your ability to obtain restorative sleep for many reasons. Discuss your medications with your physician to see if they may be contributing to insomnia.

Monitor Light Exposure

Melatonin is a naturally occurring hormone in the brain that promotes sleep. Light, including both sunlight and artificial light, suppresses the release of melatonin, causing us to feel more awake. Bright light early in the morning is a helpful way to wake up and shake off sleep. It is helpful to reduce light exposure one hour before bedtime, including turning off all screens and dimming the lights, so that melatonin can be released.

Get Regular Exercise

There is a reciprocal relationship between physical activity and sleep. Consistent daily exercise is linked with deeper, longer, better quality sleep, and getting a good night's sleep is linked to more physical exertion the next day. Exercise alone has been shown to have strong positive effects on mental health (such as reduced depression and anxiety). Building this cyclical relationship can lead to a multitude of mental and physical health benefits. The timing of exercise is also important, however, as physical exertion too close to bedtime can disrupt the body's ability to initiate sleep. Aim to do your workout at least two to three hours before bedtime.

WHY DOES ALCOHOL IMPACT SLEEP?

Some people believe that the relaxing effects of alcohol help them sleep more soundly. Sleep researcher and neuroscientist Matthew Walker is an expert on why the opposite is true. In *Why We Sleep*, he explains that alcohol is a central nervous system depressant and works by sedating the brain. The prefrontal cortex of the frontal lobe is the first area impacted by alcohol. This is the part of the brain responsible for restraint and controlling our impulses, so when it is sedated by alcohol, we experience the initial feelings of well-being and letting loose. Over the course of an evening of drinking, the impact of alcohol on the brain causes us to feel more tired, but, as Walker states, alcohol-induced sleep is not natural sleep, as evidenced by altered electrical brainwave activity. Alcohol disrupts the structure of our sleep and reduces the amount of time we can achieve both REM and slow-wave deep sleep. Even moderate-to-light drinking can cause more arousals during the night—awakenings we may not be aware of. Finally, alcohol's relaxing effects can loosen muscles, including those of your airway, which can increase snoring and is especially concerning for those individuals with sleep apnea.

Eat Wisely and Eat Less Sugar

Diets heavy in carbohydrates, especially sugar, are associated with less deep sleep and more frequent awakenings, so monitoring sugar intake and lowering your intake if it is high is a good idea. You can also time your last meal so that it promotes restorative sleep. It's better to avoid heavy meals close to bedtime and aim to feel neither too hungry nor too full before bed. If you are in the habit of snacking right before bed, you may want to keep the snack on the smaller side and avoid things like soda, candy, cookies, chocolate, ice cream, or other high-sugar foods.

Create a Calming Bedtime Ritual

Practicing a calming bedtime routine every night helps your body and mind unwind. Your bedtime routine can include reading, meditating, or any activity that feels calming, settling, and pleasant. A warm bath can also be especially helpful. After getting out of the bath, our core body temperature tends to cool quickly, and a decrease in core temperature enables the body to initiate sleep.

EXERCISE: GET STARTED

Pick one to three sleep hygiene strategies and give yourself a full day and night to practice them. Pick ones that feel doable—changes you are 100 percent willing to try and can fully commit to. Write about your experiences here. What did you learn, and what will be helpful going forward? Keep in mind that this is just a starting point. You may not see improvements immediately, and there is likely to be some trial and error as you make changes.

THE PAVLOV CONNECTION: STIMULUS CONTROL THERAPY*

Stimulus control therapy (SCT) is a behavioral program that aims to reduce conditioned arousal. As discussed earlier, being in a state of arousal is incompatible with sleep. With SCT, the bed becomes a cue for sleep, and the association between the bed and other activities or states (like anxiety or alertness) is weakened. Per SCT, you should pair the bed with sleep, and only sleep, again and again until you train your brain that the bed is for sleep and not for work, stress, planning, worrying, or tossing and turning. According to a 2006 review in the journal *Sleep*, of 37 insomnia treatment studies, there is strong evidence that SCT is a very effective component of CBT-I, and it works well in combination with other sleep hygiene practices and sleep restriction therapy.

Here are some step-by-step instructions for SCT:

1. Go to sleep when you are sleepy.
2. Use the bed only for sleep and sexual activity.
3. If you find yourself unable to sleep within about 10 to 20 minutes, get up and go to another room if possible. Stay up for as long as you wish or until you feel sleepy. While awake and out of the bedroom, do something pleasant or slightly boring (not

* Adapted from "Stimulus Control Therapy," by Richard R. Bootzin and Michael L. Perlis, in *Behavioral Treatments for Sleep Disorders: A Comprehensive Primer of Behavioral Sleep Medicine Interventions*, edited by Michael Perlis, Mark Aloia, and Brett Kuhn.

activating or stimulating) until you feel sleepy, such as reading, doing a crossword, folding laundry, or meditating. Keep the lights low. Do not work on the computer or use blue-light powered screens. When you are ready, return to bed. Do not sleep in another room.

4. If you do not fall asleep quickly (within about 10 to 20 minutes, or even sooner if you want to get out of bed because you feel anxious or frustrated), repeat step 3. Do this as many times as necessary throughout the night.

5. Get up at the same time each morning regardless of how much sleep you got the night before. Having a consistent wake-up time supports your internal clock and the creation of a reliable sleep rhythm.

6. Do not nap during the day.

MAKING SLEEP EFFICIENT: SLEEP RESTRICTION THERAPY

Sleep restriction therapy (SRT) was introduced over 30 years ago by Dr. Arthur Spielman and his colleagues and is particularly useful for those struggling with broken, fragmented, or fitful sleep. Sleep restriction is based on Spielman's 3P Model of Insomnia, which suggests that insomnia develops due to:

- Predisposing factors (such as genetic or biological vulnerabilities)
- Precipitating factors (such as a stressful event or change, like a new job or an injury)
- Perpetuating factors (such as poor sleep hygiene habits, like sleeping in, tossing and turning in bed, or worrying and catastrophizing about sleep)

SRT works by condensing the time a person is in bed to the average hours they are *actually* asleep. The treatment aims to reduce unwanted awake time in bed and capitalizes on mild sleep deprivation to help consolidate sleep. The goal is for more continuous, deeper sleep with shorter sleep onset latency (less time to fall asleep) and fewer nighttime awakenings, or better *sleep efficiency*. In other words, the less time you spend in bed awake, and the more time you spend in bed actually sleeping, the more efficient your sleep. You may remember from chapter 3 (page 37) that sleep efficiency is:

$$(TA \div TIB) \times 100\%$$

For example, imagine that Nate (whose story appeared at the beginning of this chapter) is spending an average of eight and a half hours in bed (10 p.m. to 6:30 a.m.). However, he is only sleeping about six hours at night. His sleep efficiency is relatively low:

$$(6 \text{ hours} \div 8.5 \text{ hours}) \times 100\% = 70.5\%$$

In SRT, Nate shortens his time in bed to only six hours (for example, 12:30 a.m. to 6:30 a.m.), and as his sleep deepens and consolidates and his sleep efficiency improves, he gradually increases his time spent in bed (in 15- or 30-minute increments) until he reaches his sleep time goal.

The basic instructions for SRT follow. As you will see, your sleep logs will come in handy.

1. Use at least a week of sleep logs to calculate your average actual *time asleep* (TA), your average *time in bed* (TIB), and your *sleep efficiency*. If your sleep efficiency is less than 90 percent (or less than 85 percent for older adults), and/or your sleep is restless and nonrestorative, SRT may be helpful.
2. If sleep efficiency is less than optimal, restrict your time in bed to your average time asleep.
3. Do not nap.
4. Once you have a sleep efficiency of 90 percent or more for a week, increase your time in bed by 15 to 30 minutes.
5. Repeat step 4, increasing your time in bed by 15 to 30 minutes per week as sleep efficiency improves, until you reach your sleep time goals.

It can take several weeks of SRT to reach your sleep goals. Sometimes sleep efficiency improves for a couple of weeks and then dips below 90 percent. This does not mean that SRT will not work for you. If sleep starts to become fragmented again or you are awake for long stretches at night, reduce your time in bed by 15 to 30 minutes the next week, and look at other factors that may also be contributing to your insomnia, such as sleep hygiene and cognitive and emotional factors.

DECIDING WHETHER TO DO SLEEP RESTRICTION THERAPY

SRT can be used as a stand-alone treatment for insomnia, or it can be used in combination with other sleep hygiene strategies and stimulus control therapy. You have some flexibility here. If it's not clear to you whether SRT could be useful, here are some things to consider. SRT is more likely to be effective if:

- Your sleep efficiency is less than 90 percent
- Your sleep is fitful, fragmented, and nonrestorative, or you are awake for long stretches at night
- You are willing to reduce your potential amount of total sleep in the short-term in order to consolidate sleep and increase sleep in the long-term

Note: The risks of SCT and SRT are relatively limited, but consider the following issues. If getting out of bed multiple times a night is not possible for you, do not do stimulus control therapy. If you have a medical or mental health condition that is worsened by sleep deprivation, only practice SRT with the help of an experienced professional.

Do you think SRT is a good treatment option for you? If so, are you ready to jump in right away, fully, or would you rather add SRT later in the program?

ESTABLISHING HEALTHY SLEEP HABITS

Below is a sample plan for implementing the behavioral components of CBT-I within a week. You can modify it to fit your needs, using your sleep self-assessment and sleep goals as a guide. You may also choose to take things more slowly, perhaps starting first with stimulus control and some sleep hygiene strategies and adding other components in later days and weeks when you are ready.

Sunday

- Continue filling out sleep logs for this week and throughout the program. These will provide useful data about patterns and what is working.
- Set a fixed wake-up time, using whatever time works for your schedule. Get out of bed quickly when the alarm goes off.
- Pick at least one or two sleep hygiene strategies (see pages 45 to 47) to practice, like reducing caffeine or turning off screens an hour before bed.

Monday Continue the practices you started yesterday. In addition:

- Start stimulus control therapy (see pages 48 to 49). If napping has been part of your routine, identify some alternative activities that are likely to be stimulating or stress relieving and that are not likely to induce sleepiness.
- If you have decided that sleep restriction therapy (see pages 49 to 51) would be useful and you are ready and willing to try it, reduce the number of hours you are in bed to the average number of hours you are actually asleep. For example, if you currently sleep about six hours a night, and your set wake-up time is 6:30 a.m., your bedtime this week will be 12:30 a.m. If this feels too difficult, you may hold off on this step and just start with sleep hygiene and stimulus control strategies.

Tuesday Continue the practices listed above and:

- Set up your sleep environment for sleep. Set the thermostat to 65 degrees Fahrenheit or a temperature that is cool but comfortable. Purchase earplugs if noise is an issue. Change bedding if you are too warm or too cool.

Wednesday Continue the practices listed above and:

- Create a calming bedtime ritual. As part of this, consider a warm bath or shower before bed to help initiate sleep. Also reduce light exposure, especially blue light from LED lightbulbs and screens.

Thursday Continue the practices listed above and:

- Make a weekly exercise plan and start moving. Aim to work out at least two to three hours before bedtime.

Friday Continue the practices listed above and:

- Begin to eat in a way that promotes sleep. Reduce sugar if your sugar consumption is high. Avoid heavy meals close to bedtime. Aim to go to bed sated but not uncomfortably full.

Saturday Continue the practices listed above and:

- Address any remaining sleep hygiene issues that may be impacting your sleep.
- Review your sleep logs for the week and reflect on what is working, what has been challenging, and what you want to problem-solve.
- Make a plan to continue these practices over the coming weeks in order to build the habit.

FIVE HOURS MINIMUM

You should not restrict your time in bed to less than five hours, even if you are getting less than an average of five hours of sleep. The minimum amount of time in bed should be five to five and a half hours. You can restrict sleep time by going to bed later, getting up earlier, or a little of both. Choose a strategy based on what you think would be easiest for you. Set this as your sleep schedule for one week, meaning you will go to bed at the same time and wake at the same time every day for a week. Keep in mind that this will likely lead to a short-term decrease in the amount of sleep you are getting. This decrease in sleep can be challenging, but the idea is short-term deprivation for longer-term improvement in quality of sleep and increased length of sleep.

EXERCISE: ACCEPTING SLEEPLESSNESS

As discussed earlier, battling against sleeplessness tends to push sleep further away. Cultivating an acceptance of sleeplessness in the moment is one way to increase the likelihood that sleep will come to you, naturally. It's important to note that acceptance does not mean liking or approving of. Rather, acceptance is about clearly seeing how things are and reducing the unnecessary suffering that comes from the battle. Mindfulness is a useful tool that helps people cultivate a nonjudgmental, compassionate awareness of what is happening in the present moment. With mindful awareness, you can choose what to pay attention to or where to direct your focus. The following exercise is designed to help you shift your perspective from what there is to dislike or fret about to what there is to enjoy or appreciate in the moment. You will use your senses to help you move into appreciation mode. This exercise is brief and can be used at any time you find yourself awake when you would rather be asleep.

1. Notice any thoughts you are having about being awake. These thoughts are okay. No need to change them or push them away. Let them be.

2. Bring your awareness to your breathing. This is a way to focus your attention on the present moment. You are breathing. Just watch the breath for several breath cycles. Imagine that the breath is relaxing your body and mind.

3. Now ask yourself, what is there to appreciate in this moment? What are your senses telling you? If you are in bed, you might notice the feel of the sheets on your skin. You might notice the soothing rhythm of your breathing. You might notice the quiet of nighttime. Or you might notice and tune into sounds. You might notice stillness. You might notice that there is nothing you need to do right now—you are free of obligations.

4. As you notice what there is to appreciate, simply allow yourself to experience it. Let the appreciation sink in a bit. Feel whatever feelings arise with the noticing. Then return your focus to your breathing. You can continue to focus on the breath until you are ready to end the exercise.

WHEN LIFE HAS OTHER PLANS

This program is about building habits that will support deep, restorative sleep for the long-term. However, that doesn't mean that you will have to do *everything* that is recommended in this book *forever*. There is significant variation in what people need to do to obtain enough good quality sleep. For example, sometimes after a period of insomnia has resolved, an individual may experiment with a more flexible schedule that includes occasional naps or sleeping in on weekends. Other people may find that a consistent sleep routine is so helpful that they want to stick to it to minimize disruptions. There is no one-size-fits-all approach here.

Additionally, perfectionism is not the goal when trying to build new habits. Commitment to making changes and compassion for yourself when things go awry tends to be more helpful and motivating than harsh self-criticism. There will be a necessary element of experimentation as you start making changes. Seeing this program as a process with some trial and error built in will help you learn what works and what doesn't and how to stay motivated, even if things aren't going smoothly. It is also expected that life will get in the way at times. Stressful situations like family or work obligations, illness, schedule disruptions, and unexpected events may knock you off-track. Try to see those challenges as temporary setbacks and opportunities for learning rather than total failures. And even total failures can be useful—these experiences provide lots of insightful data that you can use to try again. Sometimes you will have to revise the plan. Sometimes you may need to go back to the basics and start again. Progress is rarely a straight shot to the end goal, but rather, a journey that involves noticing when you have gotten off-track and choosing to take the steps to get back on the path.

REDUCING SCREEN TIME

Screens are ubiquitous these days, and late-night exposure to TV, computer, smart-phone, and tablet screens is extremely common. However, the light that comes from these screens can be really disruptive to sleep. That's because the blue-dominant light from screens and LED lightbulbs is especially stimulating and good at suppressing melatonin release. Reducing this blue-light exposure at night is one very helpful thing to add to your bedtime ritual. To reduce the negative impact of light on your sleep, turn off the screens and dim the lights one hour before bed. If a smartphone lives within arm's reach of your bed, you may want to find it another home. You may also want to try wearing blue-light blocking glasses in the evening and changing the settings on your smartphone and other screens to reduce the amount of blue-dominant light that is emitted in the hours before bed. If you like to read in bed, reading an actual book would be much better than reading on a device. And, if you are practicing SCT, pick a cozy spot other than the bed to read and then transition to your bed for lights out.

ASSESSMENT REVISITED

Once you have completed the first week, it will be helpful to review and track your changes, progress, and challenges. You can start by completing the "Weekly Sleep Log Summary." Here is Nate's example, as well as a blank copy. You can find extra copies of the log in the Blank Worksheets and Forms section at the end of this book (see page 111), or online at www.CallistoMediaBooks.com/InsomniaWorkbook.

SAMPLE WEEKLY SLEEP LOG SUMMARY

Nate's example

Week #: ___1___

Dates: ___2-3-19 to 2-9-19___

Average Sleep Onset Latency: ___20 minutes___

Average Estimated Time Asleep (TA): ___5.5 hours___

Average Time in Bed (TIB): ___6 hours___

Average Sleep Efficiency: (TA ÷ TIB × 100%) ___(5.5 ÷ 6.0) × 100 = 91.6___ %

Average number of awakenings: ___1.6___

Average fatigue: ___6.4___

Average quality of sleep: ___6___

Average stress/distress: ___4___

Average pain/discomfort: ___1___

WEEKLY SLEEP LOG SUMMARY

Week #: _____

Dates: _____

Average Sleep Onset Latency: _____

Average Estimated Time Asleep (TA): _____

Average Time in Bed (TIB): _____

Average Sleep Efficiency: ([TA ÷ TIB] × 100%) = _____%

Average number of awakenings: _____

Average fatigue: _____

Average quality of sleep: _____

Average stress/distress: _____

Average pain/discomfort: _____

What did you learn this week? Where have you made progress? What changes were difficult? What was easier than expected? What were the roadblocks you encountered, and how might you do it differently next week?

_____

_____

_____

_____

_____

_____

_____

MOVING FORWARD

This week focused on the behavioral components of CBT-I, including the various sleep hygiene strategies, stimulus control therapy, and sleep restriction therapy. You were given a sample plan to implement these strategies, and you can adapt that sample plan to meet your specific sleep needs and goals. You also read about (and hopefully had a chance to practice) an acceptance and appreciation exercise. Finally, you were asked to reflect on your progress so far. The next chapter will explore the cognitive components of CBT-I, help you identify how thoughts, beliefs, and attitudes may be impacting your sleep, and give you multiple tools with which you can experiment.

Hush

Zzzzz   Sleepy?   Zzzz   Sleepy?

Sleep...   NAP   Sleep...

DREAM ✳   DREAM

p...   Zzz Sleep... Z

DREAM   NAP   DREAM

Hush

Zzzzz   Zzzzz   Sleepy?

Sleepy?   NAP   Sleep...

Sleep...

DREAM ✳   DREAM

Zzz Sleep...   Z

DREAM   NAP   DREAM

UNTHINKING YOUR WAY TO SLEEP

THIS WEEK WE WILL EXPLORE the cognitive components of CBT-I. This chapter will discuss the relationship between difficult internal experiences (including thoughts and emotions) and insomnia. It focuses on strategies like noticing and changing your relationship with thoughts and beliefs, challenging unhelpful thinking and attitudes, and working effectively with negativity, anxiety, worry, and other emotions. The goal of this chapter is to give you more active cognitive coping tools and opportunities to experiment with them.

NO MORE SLEEPLESS NIGHTS

Rachel has been working hard to improve her sleep habits. She has cleaned up her nighttime routine, reduced her caffeine use, started exercising most mornings, and now has a consistent bedtime and waketime. However, she is continuing to have difficulty falling asleep, and this is making her life really difficult, as is her growing anxiety and worry.

Rachel is a new teacher and wants to do a good job. She worries about her job performance often. She describes herself as someone who is "hardwired for anxiety," and her anxiety has really impacted her quality of life on multiple occassions. She is currently in the middle of one of those periods. She feels on edge during the workday, and at night she worries about what is in store for her the next day at work, but also about bigger, scarier things. It's as if her mind goes searching for things to worry about. It's easy for Rachel to catastrophize or consider the worst-case scenario (even if it's highly unlikely to happen).

To make matters worse, Rachel is now also worrying about her lack of sleep. As she lies awake, she often thinks about impending crushing fatigue and how bad her performance will be the next day. She worries about whether this insomnia is impacting her health in the long-term. She also feels that she tends to be more anxious when she hasn't slept well, like she is in a vicious anxiety-insomnia cycle. She wants to work on breaking this cycle and is eager to learn strategies to cope better with her anxiety so that it has less impact on her sleep and her ability to enjoy her life.

RECOGNIZE YOUR STORIES ABOUT SLEEPLESSNESS

It is common for distressing stories about not sleeping to develop as insomnia lingers. Sleep is important, and fear about not sleeping increases the chance that we are going to think about sleep often. Distressing thoughts about sleep can strongly influence our emotional state, and vice versa. Our thinking can also become habitual. Sometimes we aren't even totally aware of our thinking and how it is impacting us. It's incredibly useful to begin to notice what your mind is telling you about sleep and lack of sleep. Once you have an awareness of your thoughts, you can start to see them for what they are and begin to distance yourself from them, get curious about them, start to work with them, or challenge them. Here are some common examples of distressing thoughts that occur when someone is struggling with insomnia. See if any of these sound familiar:

- "I will never get to sleep tonight."
- "I cannot handle another night like this."
- "I have to sleep right now."

- "I need to work harder to get to sleep."
- "Tomorrow is going to be terrible because I am still awake."
- "I won't be able to sleep because I am _____ (too anxious, upset, stressed, or overtired)."
- "If I can just get to sleep in the next thirty minutes, maybe tomorrow won't be a disaster."
- "I cannot function without at least eight hours of sleep."
- "I was awake all night."
- "My mood is awful when I don't sleep."
- "I'm going to have to cancel plans, again."
- "Not sleeping is hurting/damaging/destroying me."

Don't worry: These kinds of thoughts are normal. It is reasonable for you to be concerned by the fact that you are not sleeping as much as you want. It's also normal to feel distressed, anxious, fearful or frustrated by insomnia. And, while these thoughts and feelings are neither bad nor unusual, they are likely contributing to the insomnia cycle. Thoughts, beliefs, and emotions are one of the perpetuating factors that keep insomnia going. The next section will give you a variety of strategies that will help you reduce any negative impacts your thoughts and emotions may be having on your sleep. It will also give you strategies to cope better with and reduce emotional distress.

What thoughts keep you up at night? What are your distressing thoughts about sleep?

EXERCISE: WHAT ARE YOU THINKING RIGHT NOW?*

Our brains are thinking machines. We spend so much time thinking, planning, problem-solving, daydreaming, remembering, ruminating, fantasizing, and worrying. It is easy to get caught up in our own thoughts, often with little awareness of what we are thinking. To increase your awareness of your thoughts, take three minutes and write them down as they pass through your mind, while they are happening, in the space provided below.

What happened? How many thoughts were you able to catch and write down? Did you notice other thoughts or judgments about your thoughts? Did writing down your thoughts change your experience of them?

* Adapted from *Get Out of Your Mind and Into Your Life: The New Acceptance and Commitment Therapy*, by Steven C. Hayes and Spencer Smith.

CHANGING THE IMPACT OF THOUGHTS

CBT involves looking at how our thoughts, behaviors, and actions are interrelated, and the "I" includes some strategies specific to insomnia, including sleep hygiene, stimulus control, and sleep restriction discussed in week 1 (see pages 44 to 47). At the beginning of week 2 (pages 62 to 63), we discussed how fear about not sleeping can lead to unhelpful thoughts that actually push sleep further away. Below are some strategies for coping with these types of thoughts and beliefs.

"I Am Having the Thought . . ."

When you notice distressing thoughts, say out loud or silently to yourself: "I'm having the thought that . . ." Then describe the thought you are having. This is an easy way to notice and get some distance from your thoughts so that you can see them clearly, and as *just thoughts*. At the beginning of the chapter you read about Rachel, who was having many thoughts about not sleeping and what not sleeping would lead to. She was predicting the worst-case scenario about the next day's events. Examples of catastrophic thoughts are:

- "Tomorrow is going to be a disaster because I'll be so tired."
- "I'm going to screw up at work, my boss is going to see I'm not performing well, and I'm going to get fired."
- "My sleep is never going to get better, and it will probably get worse."

"Thank You, Mind"

Another way to create some distance from thoughts and potentially reduce distress is to thank your mind when it is bombarding you with worries, catastrophic thoughts, or annoying opinions. Your mind is just doing what it needs to do: It is a thinking machine, and it is wired to try and keep you safe. But sometimes the thoughts are just not helpful, like when you are worried about something you cannot control in the wee hours of the morning. So, you can say out loud or in your mind: "Thank you, mind! You are doing a great job worrying!"

Catch It, Challenge It, Change It

With this strategy, practice catching the distressing thought, challenging it by checking for accuracy, and, if the thought is distorted or unrealistic, changing it to something less distressing and less distorted. To help with reality testing, look at the following table for descriptions of common types of distorted thinking.

COMMON COGNITIVE DISTORTIONS*

Type of Distortion	Examples
All-or-nothing thinking: Looking at things in absolute, black-and-white terms.	"I got *no* sleep last night!" (when you did in fact sleep, although not as much or as well as you want)
Overgeneralization: Seeing a negative event as a never-ending pattern of defeat.	"I'm awake again, I'll never have normal sleep." "This always happens to me, and will never get better."
Mind-reading: Assuming people are reacting badly to you when there is no direct evidence.	"Pedro still hasn't responded to my email, he must be upset with me."
Fortune-telling: Predicting that things will turn out badly or catastrophizing.	"Tomorrow will be a disaster." "I won't be able to function at all." "I won't sleep tonight." "I'm going to have to cancel plans, again."
Magnifying or minimizing: Blowing things out of proportion or shrinking their significance.	"Not sleeping is destroying me!" (magnifying) "This small improvement in my sleep doesn't matter" or "That success at work is not really important." (minimizing)
Personalization and blame: You blame yourself for something for which you weren't entirely responsible.	"I need to work harder to get to sleep." "This is all my fault."
Labeling: Identifying with your shortcomings.	"I'm a jerk;" "I'm worthless;" "I'm a loser."
Should statements: Judging yourself and the situation with "I should, have to, need to, or must."	"I must sleep tonight!" "I should be asleep already."

* Adapted from *The Feeling Good Handbook* by David D. Burns.

What types of cognitive distortions do you notice in your own thinking?

_____

_____

_____

WORKING WITH YOUR NEGATIVITY BIAS

The human brain is wired to notice, look for, pay attention to, and remember the bad things that happen to us more than the positive experiences. This is called the negativity bias. It is our mind's way of trying to keep us safe from harm by helping us think about the bad things that could happen and have happened to minimize future risks and danger. But it does not help us feel content, happy, or at ease and actually keeps us from fully recognizing, taking in, or enjoying the good things that do happen. It can also keep us from doing the stuff that helps good things occur. It's a bummer! But, there are things you can do to counteract this bias toward the negative. For instance, the Three Good Things practice, developed by Dr. Martin Seligman at the University of Pennsylvania, is a short, simple exercise that has been shown to increase levels of happiness and decrease depression after one week of practice.

You might consider incorporating this practice into your evening routine. Every day for at least a week, write down three good things that happened **and** why they happened. The good things can be very small, tiny even. It could be having a pleasant interaction with a coworker, seeing something funny on YouTube, enjoying a good walk or meal, playing with your dog, watching the sunset, or hugging your kid. It can be anything, really, that was positive. The second part, the why it happened, also seems to be important. Maybe you had a good walk because you scheduled it during your lunch break, or maybe you had a pleasant interaction because you decided to say hello to your coworker. This practice helps you notice good things and increase your sense of agency and your awareness of what increases the chances of good things happening.

Write down three good things that happened today and *why*:

1.

2.

3.

DESIGNATED WORRY TIME*

Designated worry time (DWT) is a useful practice if you are noticing that worrying is frequently impacting your sleep. It was developed to help people with generalized anxiety or excessive worrying. This may seem counterintuitive, but bringing worries to mind on purpose and really *allowing* yourself to worry can cause worries to decrease in frequency and become less distressing over time. DWT works because it teaches you to delay, condense, and limit when and where you worry. It also fosters a sense of control over the feeling. This practice also uses stimulus control concepts: You are retraining your brain to understand that bed is *not* a place to worry. Here are the basic instructions:

1. **Schedule a daily time to worry for 10 to 30 minutes:** This is your designated worry time. Pick a place outside of the bedroom that is not used for work or relaxation to worry.

2. **During your scheduled worry time, only worry:** You can do this by writing out your worries, or just by bringing them to mind and *really* worrying about them, one by one. Allow yourself to think about the worst-case scenario. Think all the way to the end of the worry. Really lean into the worry. This may cause an increase in distress or anxiety. That is okay. The increase in distress is temporary. When you get to the end of your list of worries, if you still have time, start at the beginning and re-worry.

3. **Do not ruminate:** No thinking about past events, only think about future-based worries. Do not reassure yourself. Only worry. If solutions come to mind, you can note them and then return to worrying.

4. **Delay:** If worries come up outside of your designated worry time, delay worrying until your next scheduled session. Actively remind your mind that you *can and will worry*, but not until your next designated worry time. Tell yourself, "Okay, mind. I can worry about that, but not until my next scheduled worry session."

* Adapted from "Cognitive-Behavioural Therapy for Worry and Generalised Anxiety Disorder," by Michelle G. Newman and Thomas D. Borkovec, in *Cognitive Behaviour Therapy: A Guide for the Practising Clinician*, edited by Gregoris Simos.

PUTTING IT TOGETHER

Let's review some of the main concepts from this chapter and think about how you can incorporate some of them into your own sleep plan. It's also important to note that these strategies are not just for helping you sleep. These are life skills that can be useful for a variety of stressful situations.

Don't Fight It

Acceptance of thoughts, feelings, and difficult internal experiences is step one in lessening their negative impacts on sleep and your overall quality of life. Fighting against these experiences only adds an extra layer of suffering. Instead of trying to push thoughts or feelings away, you can label them as simply "thoughts" and bring compassion to yourself and your experience. Also remember the stimulus control concepts: If you are in bed and are feeling stressed or anxious or frustrated, get out of bed, go to another room, and use one of the strategies in this chapter to work with these thoughts and feelings.

More Than "Positive Thinking"

It can be helpful to note whether our thoughts and beliefs are helpful or unhelpful. Challenging distorted or catastrophic thinking sometimes reduces distress. But the idea is not to force yourself to have happy thoughts. Trying to force happiness doesn't really work. Plus, you don't need to be happy for sleep to arrive. Again, you can gently challenge unhelpful thoughts or simply acknowledge them, let them be, and redirect your attention. This idea of redirecting attention will be discussed in more detail in week 3 in the "Exploring Mindfulness, Meditation, and Relaxation" section (page 76).

Make Time to Process

In addition to scheduling designated worry time (see page 68) and using the "Working with Your Negativity Bias" exercise (page 67), it can be helpful to carve out some time at the end of the day just to process and mentally decompress. This is especially helpful if you are very busy and have little downtime during the day to just be alone with your thoughts. Making a to-do list for tomorrow, spending some time journaling about your day, or talking with a friend or partner are ways to do this. You can experiment with the timing, but aim to have some space between processing and getting into bed. The idea, again, is to do this mental work *before* you get into bed. Then, if worrying, ruminating, or problem-solving starts when you are in bed, you can gently remind yourself that your work for today is done and you'll start again tomorrow.

Assessment Revisited

Once you have completed week 2 of the program, it's once again helpful to pause and review. You can start by completing the "Weekly Sleep Log Summary" for this week. Here is Rachel's example as well as a blank log. (You may recall from the beginning of the chapter that Rachel has been working on her sleep hygiene and has begun applying cognitive tools this week to help with her stress and anxiety.) You can find extra copies of the log in the Blank Worksheets and Forms section at the end of this book (see page 111) or online at www.CallistoMediaBooks.com/InsomniaWorkbook.

SAMPLE WEEKLY SLEEP LOG SUMMARY

Rachel's example:

Week #: ___2___

Dates: ___2-3-19 to 2-9-19___

Average Sleep Onset Latency: ___30 minutes___

Average Estimated Time Asleep (TA): ___7 hours___

Average Time in Bed (TIB): ___8 hours___

Average Sleep Efficiency: ([TA ÷ TIB] × 100%) ___(7.0 ÷ 8.0) × 100 = 87.5___ %

Average number of awakenings: ___2___

Average fatigue: ___5___

Average quality of sleep: ___6___

Average stress/distress: ___3___

Average pain/discomfort: ___0___

WEEKLY SLEEP LOG SUMMARY

Week #: _____

Dates: _____

Average Sleep Onset Latency: _____

Average Estimated Time Asleep (TA): _____

Average Time in Bed (TIB): _____

Average Sleep Efficiency: ([TA ÷ TIB] × 100%) = _____%

Average number of awakenings: _____

Average fatigue: _____

Average quality of sleep: _____

Average stress / distress: _____

Average pain / discomfort: _____

What did you learn in week 2? What coping strategies did you find helpful? What do you want to practice more? What can you solve to make things easier?

_____

_____

_____

_____

_____

_____

_____

MOVING FORWARD

This week focused on strategies to increase your awareness of thoughts, help you get distance from distorted thoughts in order to see them more clearly, and reduce the negative impact thoughts might be having on your emotional state, your behaviors, and your sleep. You were given opportunities to practice observing, distancing, and challenging and changing thoughts. You also now have techniques to reduce worry and work with your brain's negativity bias. Keep practicing in order to break unhelpful patterns and build new, healthier ones. The more you practice, the less power unhelpful thoughts will have over your sleep and quality of life. During the next two weeks, we will dive deeper into mindfulness skills and discuss specific relaxation tools and complementary approaches. You will also get a chance to create your individualized sleep plan.

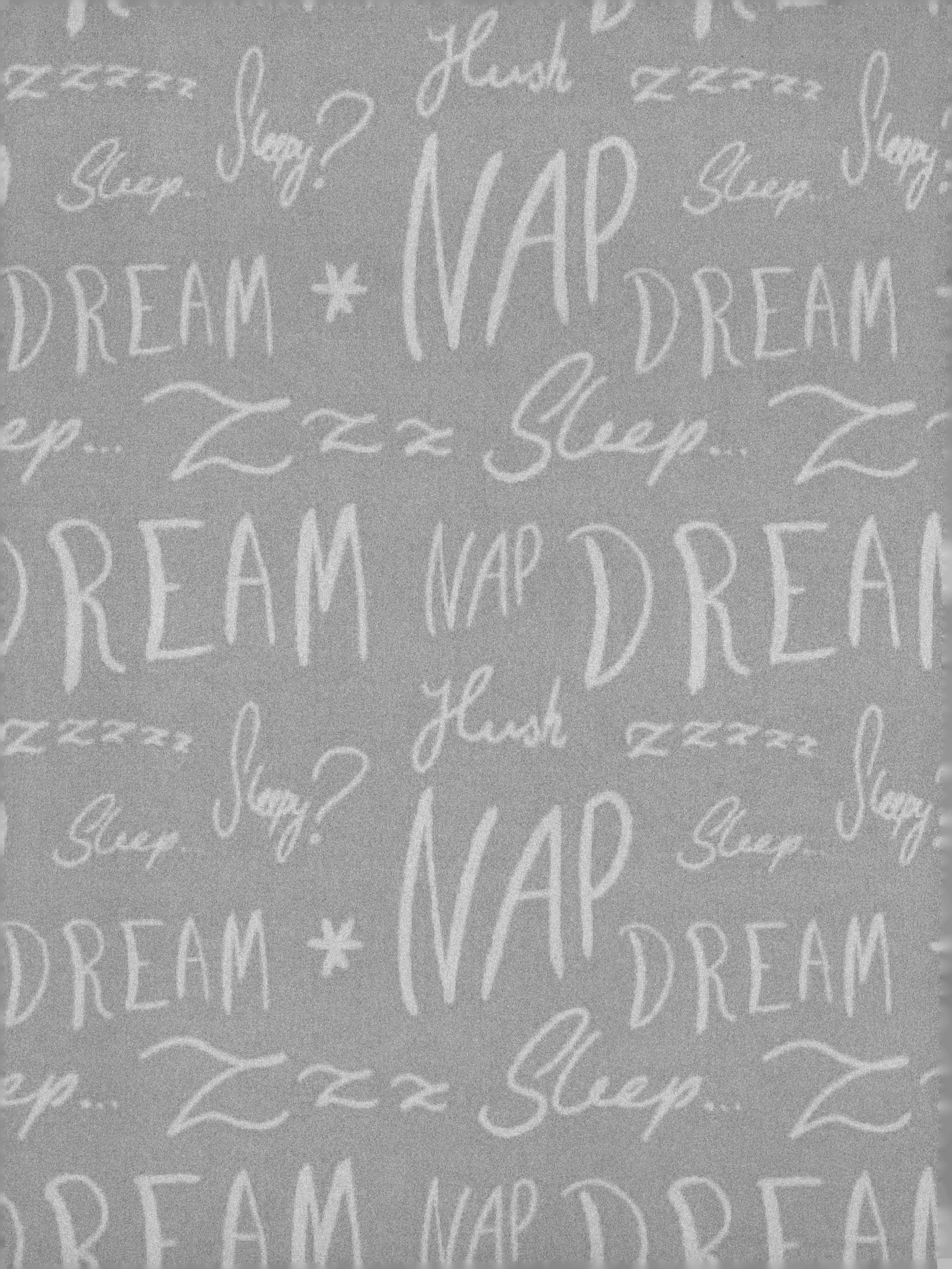
Hush
Zzzzz
Sleepy?
Sleep...
NAP
DREAM
Zzz
Sleep...
NAP
DREAM

RELAXING INTO SLEEP

THIS WEEK WE WILL EXPLORE EXERCISES that can help reduce stress and activate your body's natural relaxation response. These are exercises that you can practice during the day for general stress management, before bed as part of a nightly wind-down routine, or if you are having difficulty in the middle of the night. We will focus on general relaxation techniques, as well as mindfulness and meditation strategies.

NO MORE SLEEPLESS NIGHTS

Isaiah had back surgery two years ago that corrected some issues with his spine, but he still experiences pain that impacts his sleep, his mood, and his activity level. He has a difficult time getting comfortable and staying comfortable in bed. Most nights he wakes up due to discomfort and moves to his recliner or the couch to try to sleep there instead. His sleep is fitful and fragmented.

Isaiah has started working on improving his sleep by practicing good sleep hygiene habits, like reducing his caffeine and alcohol consumption. He has also reduced his late-night light exposure by turning off his computer an hour before bed and not looking at his cell phone. He is working hard, and his sleep is improving. He is falling asleep more quickly. However, pain and related stress and anxiety are continuing to keep him from restorative sleep. Now when he wakes up in the middle of the night due to pain, his mind latches on to negative thoughts that push sleep further away. He's just started to use cognitive coping strategies like challenging negative thoughts and worries about lack of sleep, and he has plans to continue to build these skills.

Don't worry if you feel like Isaiah does. There is hope, because, like Isaiah, you are now ready to try relaxation and mindfulness tools that are particularly useful for reducing the negative impacts of pain and physical discomfort. Let's learn more about these practices together.

EXPLORING MINDFULNESS, MEDITATION, AND RELAXATION

In chapter 2, you were introduced to the concepts of mindfulness, acceptance, and relaxation and how they are useful in helping you set the stage for sleep (see pages 18 to 19). During this week of the program, we will explore mindfulness and relaxation techniques in more depth. You will be given many practical suggestions and formal exercises that will teach you more about fostering calm and relaxation to set the stage for more restorative sleep.

Mindfulness

Mindfulness is about paying attention to the present moment in a way that is compassionate and nonjudgmental. It's about noticing and accepting what is happening so that you can work with whatever is happening in a wise and intentional way. As we have discussed, fighting against sleeplessness pushes sleep further away. The "Accepting Sleeplessness" exercise (page 54) is an example of a mindfulness practice that is about letting go of

EXERCISE: MINDFUL BREATH MEDITATION

Below are instructions for a classic mindful breath meditation. While it can be used at any time, let's focus on making it a part of your calming nighttime ritual. You can do this in bed, but if you are doing stimulus control therapy, limit the amount of time you practice this in bed. Remember, in SCT, the bed should be for just sleep and sex. If you are awake in the middle of the night and doing SCT, you can practice this breath meditation outside of bed as your calming activity to do until you feel sleepy. If you are a beginner, you may want to record yourself reading this meditation and use the audio as a guide at first.

1. Start by settling in. Close your eyes if that is comfortable; if not, simply soften your gaze and pick a spot to focus on.
2. Take an upright position with your neck and back straight but not rigid. Or lie down in a way that feels comfortable.
3. Place your hands wherever they are comfortable.
4. Bring awareness to your body. Notice the contact of your body with the chair, bed, or floor. Invite your body to begin to relax, to let go of any stress or tension that has been building today.
5. Become aware that your body is breathing. There is no need to change the breath. Just notice the breath wherever you feel it and use the breath as an anchor. When you notice that you've become distracted or lost in thought, be compassionate with yourself. This is normal. You do not need to clear your mind or try to stop thinking. Instead, gently notice that your mind has drifted and bring your awareness back to your breathing.
6. Bring your awareness back to your breath again and again. This noticing and coming back to the breath is the practice. If you like, you can set a timer for the length of time you would like to meditate. Or, when you are ready to bring the exercise to an end, simply open your eyes.

struggling against sleeplessness. Mindfulness practices can be formal like this or they can be informal acts, like bringing mindful awareness to eating, walking, or any other activity. For example, taking a shower mindfully could involve simply paying attention to sensations while showering: the warmth of the water, the smell of soap, and the restorative effects of the heat. Mindfully drinking a cup of decaffeinated tea could also be a nighttime ritual. I've also listed some books and apps for mindfulness in the Resources section at the end of the book (see page 113).

Relaxation Strategies

The relaxation response, a term coined by Dr. Herbert Benson, consists of physiological processes or changes that are the opposite of the body's stress or fight-or-flight response. You can think of these strategies as ways to turn down or recover from the stress response and return to a state of rest. As we have discussed, sleep is a state of relative inactivity. In contrast, stress is a state of activation and cognitive and physiological arousal. When stress and arousal are reduced, it is easier to fall asleep and stay asleep. We also know that there tends to be cyclical relationships between stress, emotional distress, pain, and sleep, with each factor potentially impacting or exacerbating the other. Turning on the relaxation response can serve to reduce pain, stress, and emotional distress, which then makes it easier to sleep. Instructions for "Progressive Muscle Relaxation" (page 83) and "Imagery and Visualization" (pages 19 to 20) exercises are given later in this section.

WORKING WITH PAIN AND PHYSICAL DISCOMFORT

Sometimes the primary reason for disrupted sleep is pain or other physical discomfort. Often this discomfort is due to a temporary condition, such as pregnancy or recovery from injury. Other times, the condition is long-term or chronic. Whether acute or chronic, pain and physical discomfort should be evaluated by your physician. Some of the strategies discussed in this chapter may also help you cope. Below are some common long-term issues that can contribute to poor-quality sleep.

Chronic Pain

Chronic pain can develop for many reasons—including specific diagnoses like fibromyalgia, arthritis, complex regional pain syndrome, or back and neck problems, to name just a few. Chronic pain can take a toll on your emotional well-being, your activity level, your stress level, and your sleep. In addition, poor sleep, stress, and lack of activity can make chronic pain worse. Many of the exercises in this chapter can help you cope more effectively with chronic pain by reducing stress, distress, and tension with the goal of improving sleep. Additionally, working with your physician and other health providers to increase your activity level and exercise can help break the vicious cycles between sleep and activity level and chronic pain.

Restless Legs Syndrome

As described in chapter 3, restless legs syndrome (RLS) is characterized by a strong, irresistible urge to move your legs, typically in response to uncomfortable sensations (see page 9). RLS is primarily treated with medications and vitamins. Sometimes RLS is caused by an underlying condition that can be corrected, such as an iron deficiency. Exercise, stretching, heat, cold, massage, and good sleep hygiene may also be helpful.

Hot Flashes Associated with Menopause

Changing hormone levels during menopause can cause hot flashes in women, which are sudden feelings of intense warmth, especially in the chest, neck, and face. Hot flashes may be accompanied by sweating and chills once the hot flash ends. When this happens at night, sleep is often disrupted. Hot flashes can be treated medically or with complementary approaches like acupuncture. In addition, wearing lightweight clothing, using lightweight bedding, and avoiding spicy food, caffeine, alcohol, and nicotine near bedtime may be helpful. You may want to have a change of clothes ready if sweating from the hot flashes is heavy. Additionally, using stimulus control strategies might be useful. For example, leaving the bedroom and practicing one of the relaxation strategies in this chapter can help with recovery from the hot flash and can reduce the brain's association of the bedroom with heat and discomfort.

EXERCISE: BODY SCAN*

The body scan is another classic mindfulness practice that can help you relax the body and tune into physical sensations. This is an effective practice for developing both deep concentration and flexible attention. It typically involves lying on your back and moving your awareness through the different regions of your body, but if lying on your back is uncomfortable or not possible, you can sit upright or lie on your side. At the end of the practice, you may feel a shift in your energy level and physical and mental states. The body scan can be especially helpful if you are coping with chronic pain or other physical discomfort.

Here are the basic instructions:

1. Lie down on your back (or another position that works for you) in a comfortable place. Make sure that you are warm enough.
2. Allow your eyes to gently close. If you are doing this at a time when you want to stay awake, and staying awake is difficult, keep your eyes open, soften your gaze, and pick a spot to focus on.
3. Feel the rise and fall of your abdomen with each inbreath and outbreath.
4. Take a few moments to feel your body, from head to toe, and any sensations in the body or at points of contact with the bed or floor.
5. Bring your attention to the toes of your left foot. As you focus your attention on your toes, see if you can direct or channel your breathing to them as well, so that it feels as if you are breathing into your toes and out from your toes. This may take some practice. It may help to just imagine your breath traveling down from your nose into your lungs and then continuing through the abdomen and down the left leg all the way to the toes and then back again and out through the nose.
6. Allow yourself to notice and feel any and all sensations from your toes. If you don't feel anything at the moment, that is okay too. Just allow yourself to feel "not feeling anything."

7. When you are ready to leave the toes and move on, take a deeper, more intentional breath all the way down to the toes and, on the outbreath, allow them to "dissolve" in your mind's eye. Stay with your breathing for a few breaths and then move in turn to the sole of the foot, the heel, the top on the foot, and then the ankle, continuing to breathe into and out from each region as you observe the sensations that you are experiencing, then letting go of the sensations and moving on.

8. Each time you notice that your attention has wandered off, gently bring your mind back to the breath and to the region you are focusing on.

9. Continue to move slowly up your left leg. Then do the same for your right foot and leg. Then move through the rest of your body, one region at a time. Maintain the focus on the breath and on the sensations in each body region. Breathe into and out from each region, and then let that region go. If you are experiencing pain in a particular area, visualize or imagine the breath is softening, soothing, and easing your experience.

10. It is helpful to practice the body scan daily for at least two weeks to begin to build a solid mindfulness practice, and the body scan was originally designed to be completed in about 45 minutes. If that seems overwhelming, it is still very useful to do a shorter version (10 to 20 minutes) of the practice.

* Adapted from *Full Catastrophe Living: Using the Wisdom of Your Body and Mind to Face Stress, Pain, and Illness* by Jon Kabat-Zinn.

STRESS MANAGEMENT

A high level of stress can negatively impact sleep, and general stress management can be a useful set of tools for improving sleep. Many of the strategies we have discussed in previous chapters are recommended for stress management, such as practicing the exercises, "Working with Your Negativity Bias" (page 67), "Designated Worry Time" (page 68), and good nutrition. Mindfulness and relaxation are excellent for reducing stress over time. Let's go over some other stress management tips.

Do What You Can and Accept the Rest

Problem-solving is an effective stress management tool. If there is an identifiable problem in your life that is causing you stress, doing what you can to solve the problem can foster a sense of control, relieve some distress, and potentially make things better. Here are four steps to help solve any problem in a healthy way:

1. Identify the specific problem—clearly define the problem for yourself.
2. Generate a list of solutions, evaluate them, and select the best option.
3. Make an action plan.
4. Carry out the plan, one step at a time.

The flip side of problem-solving is acceptance. Not all problems are solvable or completely solvable. Accepting what we cannot change reduces our suffering. Remember, it is not the same as *liking* how things are, nor is it resignation. It's more about a willingness to see things as they are to reduce unnecessary struggle, pain, and frustration.

Cultivate Self-Compassion

Most of us have a self-critical part of ourselves that can exacerbate our suffering when things aren't going well. Increasing self-compassion can ease our stress and distress. You can practice cultivating your compassionate self by first noticing if what you are saying to yourself is overly harsh, judgmental, or highly critical. Then respond by giving yourself the same care and compassion you would give to a good friend. There are many resources available to help you practice self-compassion. I recommend *Self-Compassion* by Dr. Kristin Neff—one of the leading experts in this area.

EXERCISE: PROGRESSIVE MUSCLE RELAXATION

Progressive muscle relaxation (PMR) is a technique that was first developed in the 1930s by Dr. Edmund Jacobson to reduce tension and induce physiological relaxation. In this exercise, you systematically tense and release different muscle groups, paying attention to the differences in sensations of tension and relaxation. This practice is an active strategy and can be particularly helpful for those who have difficulty relaxing when sitting quietly.

1. Find a comfortable position, either sitting or lying down. Close your eyes if that is comfortable, or just pick a spot to focus on and soften your gaze.

2. Become aware of your breathing. Focus on the breath for a few moments, allowing the breath to slow a little if that feels comfortable. Notice sensations of breathing wherever you feel them.

3. Start with your right foot. On the next inbreath, tense the muscles of your right foot, perhaps by curling your toes or flexing the foot back toward your head. The tightness or level of tension you hold is up to you. Tense or squeeze the muscles in whatever way feels comfortable to you. It does not need to be painful. After tensing for a few moments, release the tension and relax your foot completely. Continue to breathe in a way that is comfortable and natural. Notice the difference in the sensations of tension and relaxation.

4. On the next inbreath, tense the muscles of the lower right leg and calf. After tensing for a few moments, release the tension and really relax the right leg. Again, pay attention to the differences in the sensations of tension and relaxation.

5. With the next inbreath, tense the muscles of the upper right leg and buttock. Hold the tension for a few moments, and when you are ready, release the tension and relax the entire right leg. Notice the difference in the sensations of tension and relaxation.

6. Repeat this sequence for the left leg. Then, progress up the body, tensing and releasing the muscle groups. Include the abdomen, chest and back, the hands and arms, the shoulders and neck, and the muscles of the face and tongue. Continue to breathe in a way that feels natural and soothing. Continue to pay attention to sensations of tension and relaxation.

7. Once you have moved through the body, return your focus to the breath for a few moments, and when you are ready, end the exercise.

Connect with Others

Humans are social animals. We need each other. Sharing our struggles with others in similar situations tends to reduce distress. Additionally, just getting together to do something you enjoy with another person is helpful for stress reduction and can give you a mood boost. If your social group is already robust, capitalize on that. If it is not, start taking steps to increase your social connections. This can include making a coffee date, joining a group, going to a church service, volunteering, or engaging in weekly calls or e-mails with friends or family members.

Get Outside

Research has shown us that being outside, in nature, reduces stress, anxiety, and depression and creates feelings of well-being. Exercising outdoors, especially in scenic settings, has added benefits over exercising in a gym. So, bike along the lake, take a walk in the woods, go hiking, or spend an afternoon at the beach when you can.

LIGHTS AND SOUNDS

If you are looking to an external way to help you sleep, there are a lot of options out there that can be used in conjunction with CBT-I. Let's go over the technology that can help you get better quality sleep.

Light Therapy

Week 1 discussed how light can impact our circadian rhythms and natural sleep-wake cycle (see page 46). The best light source is natural outdoor light. However, depending on where you live and your life and work situation, you may not have access to enough natural light when it would be most helpful. Light therapy boxes and lamps use bulbs that mimic natural outdoor light. Light therapy is sometimes used for circadian rhythm disorders. It's important to discuss light therapy with your physician before beginning. Light therapy does carry some risks and may be contraindicating in some cases, especially for individuals with bipolar disorders (it can trigger manic episodes), seizures, or migraines. Additionally, the dosage and timing of light are important variables to be discussed with your doctor, therapist, or sleep specialist.

Meditation Apps and Guided Meditations

There are many good meditation apps available, and they are generally relatively inexpensive or free. If you are just learning to meditate, an app can be useful. There is a wide range in complexity and functions of meditation apps. Some are primarily simple meditation timers and others are more complex and offer many different guided meditations which are specific to a presenting issue, like sleep or anxiety. If you do use an app, I recommend that you devote at least some time each week to meditating *without* the app or audio guidance to facilitate skill growth and autonomy and to reduce dependence on any external tools. The Resources section at the end of the book lists some recommended meditation and relaxation apps (see page 114).

Sound Machines

In week 1, we discussed the importance of having a quiet and comfortable bedroom for good quality sleep (see page 45). If noise is an issue, you can try earplugs, but you may also want to try a white or pink noise machine or app, or a fan to reduce noise.

ASSESSMENT REVISITED

It's helpful to continue to review and track changes, progress, and challenges on a weekly basis. You can start by completing the "Weekly Sleep Log Summary" below. Here is Isaiah's example as well as a blank copy. You can find extra copies of the log in the Blank Worksheets and Forms section at the end of this book (see page 111), or online at www.CallistoMediaBooks.com/InsomniaWorkbook.

SAMPLE WEEKLY SLEEP LOG SUMMARY

Isaiah's example:

Week #: _2_

Dates: _3-24-19 to 3-30-19_

Average Sleep Onset Latency: _10 minutes_

Average Estimated Time Asleep (TA): _7 hours_

Average Time in Bed (TIB): _8 hours_

Average Sleep Efficiency: ([TA ÷ TIB] × 100%) _(7.0 ÷ 8.0) × 100 = 87.5_ %

Average number of awakenings: _3_

Average fatigue: _6_

Average quality of sleep: _5_

Average stress/distress: _4_

Average pain/discomfort: _5_

WEEKLY SLEEP LOG SUMMARY

Week #: _____

Dates: _____

Average Sleep Onset Latency: _____

Average Estimated Time Asleep (TA): _____

Average Time in Bed (TIB): _____

Average Sleep Efficiency: ([TA ÷ TIB] × 100%) = _____%

Average number of awakenings: _____

Average fatigue: _____

Average quality of sleep: _____

Average stress / distress: _____

Average pain / discomfort: _____

What did you learn this week? Where have you made progress? What mindfulness, relaxation, and stress management tools do you want to continue to practice? What do you want to do differently next week?

MOVING FORWARD

We explored mindfulness and relaxation strategies to help you reduce stress and turn on the relaxation response. This week covered both formal and informal mindfulness practices, and specific relaxation exercises that you can use throughout the day and night. We explored the link between pain and discomfort and insomnia, with advice for actively coping with physical discomfort. We also discussed tips for better stress management in general, including effective problem-solving, cultivating self-compassion, connecting with others, and spending time in nature. I encourage you to experiment with exercises in this chapter and continue to practice. With continued practice, your skill level and effectiveness are likely to increase. The next chapter will review all the strategies covered in previous weeks of the program and will help you design your ongoing sleep management plan in order to build long-term habits for better, deeper, more restorative sleep.

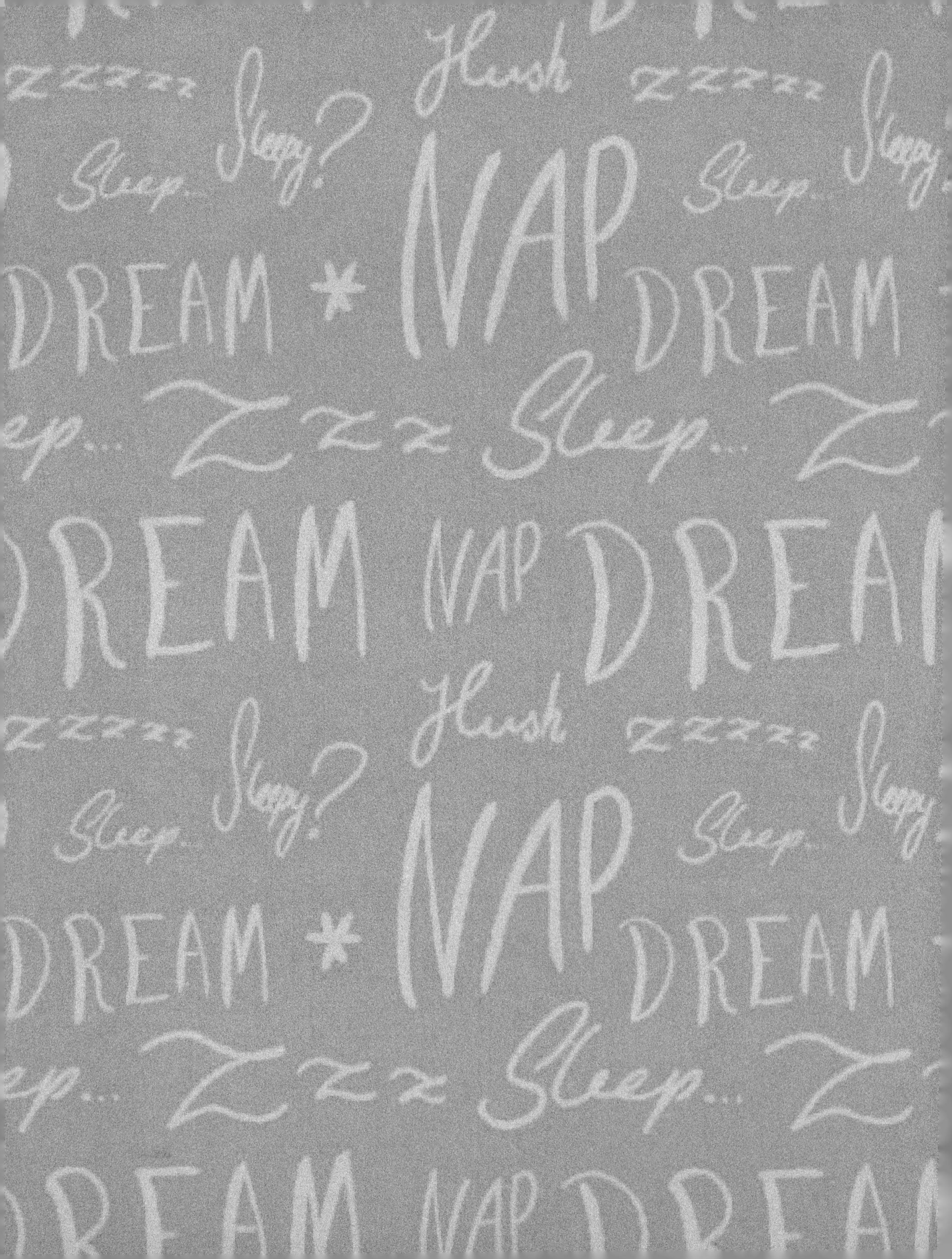
Hush
Zzzzzz
Sleepy?
Sleep...
NAP
DREAM
Zzz

MAKING A PLAN

WELCOME TO WEEK 4! So far you have completed a sleep evaluation to examine your sleep quality, quantity, patterns, and behaviors. You have also been introduced to the best interventions that CBT-I has to offer for improving your sleep. You've been invited to begin practicing behavioral and cognitive strategies to improve sleep, as well as mindfulness, relaxation, and stress management exercises.

This week is about creating your own comprehensive, individualized sleep plan based on your assessment, what you have been practicing over the last three weeks, and what you need to do to continue to make progress. This plan will include all the strategies you want to practice in order to accomplish your specific sleep goals.

NO MORE SLEEPLESS NIGHTS

Remember Greg from chapter 1 (see page 4)? He had been struggling with insomnia for many months. He had a hard time falling asleep and staying asleep. He had stopped doing many things that were important to him due to fatigue. He was worried and frustrated about not sleeping.

Imagine that Greg has spent the last three weeks practicing the various strategies in this program. His sleep logs are giving him some data that his sleep is starting to improve, he is feeling a bit more rested during the day, and his anxiety and frustration are reduced. But he knows that this is a critical moment, and that if he stops working, he is likely to revert to old, easy patterns that contribute to poor sleep. Greg wants to continue to make progress—he is committed to continuing to work toward getting better sleep. He is now ready to create his individualized sleep plan to help him stay on track to meeting his sleep goals.

BEHAVIORAL STRATEGIES: SLEEP HYGIENE, STIMULUS CONTROL, AND SLEEP RESTRICTION

The following is a checklist that includes the behavioral components of CBT-I. These were covered in week 1 (see pages 45 to 51) and include sleep hygiene strategies, stimulus control therapy, and sleep restriction therapy. Put a check next to the strategies that you want to start or continue to practice. Include the strategies that you have already incorporated into your routine, as well as those that you still want to try or currently have difficulty with. The idea is to create a list of behaviors that you can build into good sleep habits. If you have concerns or want to make notes to yourself about any of the strategies you will be practicing, write them down underneath each strategy.

○ Maintain a consistent sleep schedule.

_____

○ Reduce or eliminate naps.

_____

○ Make the sleep environment more sleep-friendly:
  ○ Lower your bedroom temperature
  ○ Change your bedding and/or mattress
  ○ Buy earplugs or a sound machine to reduce disruptive noise
  ○ Buy shades or blackout curtains

○ Reduce substance use:
  ○ Caffeine
  ○ Alcohol
  ○ Nicotine
  ○ Discuss medications with your physician to see if they may be contributing to insomnia

○ Turn off screens and dim the lights an hour before bed.

_____

○ Get bright light exposure early in the morning.

_____

○ Exercise regularly (at least 2 to 3 hours before bed).

_____

○ Avoid big meals right before bed and reduce your sugar intake.

_____

○ Create a calming bedtime ritual (describe below):

_____

_____

○ Stimulus control therapy (pages 48 to 49).

_____

○ Sleep restriction therapy (pages 49 to 51).

_____

○ Other:

_____

COGNITIVE STRATEGIES

Below is a checklist that includes the cognitive components of CBT-I that were covered in week 2 (see pages 65 to 66). Again, put a check next to the strategies that you are interested in. Include the strategies that you have already incorporated into your routine, as well as those that you still want to try or currently have difficulty with. The idea is to create a list of cognitive strategies that you will include in your individualized sleep plan. Again, write down any concerns or notes underneath each strategy.

○ Notice and label distressing thoughts in order to see them just as thoughts.

_____

○ Distance yourself from thoughts using the "I Am Having the Thought..." strategy (page 65).

_____

○ Challenge and change unhelpful thoughts.

_____

○ Distance yourself from unhelpful thoughts using the "Thank You, Mind" approach (page 65).

_____

○ Practice the "Working with Your Negativity Bias" exercise (page 67).

_____

○ Practice the "Designated Worry Time" exercise (page 68).

_____

○ Other:

_____

MINDFULNESS AND RELAXATION-BASED STRATEGIES

Below is a checklist that includes the mindfulness and relaxation strategies covered in week 3 (see pages 76 to 81). Again, put a check next to the strategies that you want to start or continue practicing, including those that may be more challenging. Write down any concerns, fears, or notes underneath each strategy.

○ "Mindful Breath Meditation" exercise (page 77).

_____

○ "Body Scan" exercise (pages 80 to 81).

_____

○ "Progressive Muscle Relaxation" exercise (page 83).

_____

○ "Imagery and Visualization" exercise (pages 19 to 20).

_____

_____

○ "Accepting Sleeplessness" exercise (page 54).

_____

○ Stress-management strategies:
    ○ Practice problem-solving and acceptance
    ○ Spend time in nature
    ○ Practice self-compassion
    ○ Connect with others

○ Other:

_____

CREATING YOUR SLEEP PLAN

Review what strategies from the previous lists have worked for you. First, we are going to look at a sample individualized sleep plan for Greg for our example. After, you are going to fill in your own sleep plan that is specific to your needs and goals. Keep in mind that this is a starting point. As you make progress toward your goals, your sleep plan may change.

Example: Greg's Individualized Sleep Plan

1. Continue stimulus control therapy.	7. Nap early and briefly, or not at all.
2. Continue sleep restriction therapy.	8. Practice the "Designated Worry Time" exercise (10 min, during lunch break).
3. Limit alcohol and sugar.	9. No caffeine after 12 p.m.
4. Maintain a calming bedtime ritual, including 20 minutes of meditation, bath, and the "Working with Your Negativity Bias" exercise.	10. Continue the "Accepting Sleeplessness" exercise.
5. Dim the lights and turn off screens 1 hr before bed.	11. Continue the "Thank you, Mind" exercise.
6. Exercise 4 to 6 times per week, 30 min.	12. Continue daily and weekly sleep logs to track progress and issues.

YOUR INDIVIDUALIZED SLEEP PLAN

Here is a blank chart you can use to create your own individualized sleep plan. Use your completed checklist from this chapter to create your specific plan.

ASSESSMENT REVISITED

It's useful to continue to complete the sleep logs as you follow your sleep plan so that you can track your progress and changes. Here is a blank "Weekly Sleep Log Summary" that you can fill out. You can find extra copies of the log in the Blank Worksheets and Forms section at the end of this book (see page 111), or online at www.CallistoMediaBooks .com/InsomniaWorkbook.

WEEKLY SLEEP LOG SUMMARY

Week #: _____

Dates: _____

Average Sleep Onset Latency: _____

Average Estimated Time Asleep (TA): _____

Average Time in Bed (TIB): _____

Average Sleep Efficiency: ([TA ÷ TIB] × 100%) = _____%

Average number of awakenings: _____

Average fatigue: _____

Average quality of sleep: _____

Average stress/distress: _____

Average pain/discomfort: _____

What have you learned over the last four weeks? Where have you made progress? Where might you need to improve?

_____

_____

_____

_____

_____

_____

_____

_____

_____

WHAT ABOUT SLEEP AIDS?

You may be taking a sleep aid occasionally or nightly. If you have been taking sleep aids consistently and want to stop, it is best to do this with the guidance of your physician. You may remember the concept of rebound insomnia from the sleep aids discussion in chapter 2 (see page 24). This is a temporary period of disrupted sleep that can sometimes occur when someone stops taking a sleep aid suddenly. It can sometimes be minimized by gradual weaning. If you experience rebound insomnia after stopping a sleep aid, that does not necessarily mean that you will never be able to sleep without a supplement or medication.

MOVING FORWARD

This week we reviewed everything covered in the last three weeks: the behavioral sleep strategies from the first week, the cognitive strategies from the second week, and the mindfulness and relaxation strategies from the third week. You've had the opportunity to reflect on what you've been practicing and what you need to do to continue making progress. You now have a comprehensive sleep plan that's specific to your sleep needs and goals. It's possible that you have made significant progress since starting the program. However, it often takes much longer than four weeks for people to reach their ultimate sleep goals. Continuing to practice and problem-solve barriers, as well as using your sleep logs to track progress, are important parts of the process of building healthy sleep habits that work for you. If you have made significant gains, congratulations! If you haven't yet seen results, or progress is going more slowly than you had hoped, do not despair. The next section lists some common problems people experience and offers tips for trouble-shooting and accessing additional support.

Zzzzz   Hush   Zzzz   Sleepy
Sleep   Sleepy?
NAP   DREAM
DREAM *
Zzz Sleep...   Z

DREAM NAP DREAM

Zzzzz   Hush   Zzzz   Sleepy
Sleep   Sleepy?
NAP   DREAM
DREAM *
Zzz Sleep...   Z

DREAM NAP DREAM

CONCLUSION

AS YOU ARRIVE AT THE END OF THIS BOOK, my hope is that you are on your way to better sleep. Over the last few weeks you have been introduced to the best that CBT-I has to offer. I want to encourage you to continue following your individualized sleep plan to build healthy sleep habits. If you find that you continue to struggle with insomnia despite your best efforts, you may also consider working with a sleep specialist. It's also recommended that you speak with your physician if you think you may need a sleep study or if you have continued concerns about your sleep or health. Read on to learn more about the specifics of sleep studies, ways to troubleshoot barriers that can get in the way of your progress, and how to access social and emotional support throughout the process.

TROUBLESHOOTING

It's now time to review your progress and see what is working, what is not, and what more is to be done. If you have not made as much progress as you would like, read below to learn about common problems and some troubleshooting ideas.

I'm Having a Hard Time Staying Awake

If you are doing sleep restriction therapy and can't seem to stay up late enough, you can consider whether going to bed earlier and getting up earlier will work better for you. Many people have an easier time staying up later than getting up earlier, but you can experiment. Another strategy is to plan out the activities you will do during the late evening hours. This might include leaving the house to read at a coffee shop or going grocery shopping, but do not drive if you are too sleepy. Avoid activities where you are likely to accidentally fall asleep.

I'm Having a Hard Time Doing Stimulus Control

Stimulus control therapy is easier when you have prepared beforehand. This includes picking the activity you are going to do when you leave the bedroom and setting it up in advance. Additionally, an important component of SCT is sticking to a set wake-up time. Getting out of bed right away, even though you may be very sleepy, and getting some bright light will signal your brain to stop releasing melatonin and help you shake off sleepiness.

I'm Not Limiting Screen Exposure

First, if your smartphone or other screen is within easy reach of your bed, move it farther away or out of the room to ease the temptation. Second, create a list of pleasant alternative activities you can do instead of being in front of a screen. You can repurpose screen time and use that time to develop a hobby, get work or tasks done, or connect with friends. Do something else that is valuable, fun, or meaningful to you.

I'm Still Napping

If you are having difficulty eliminating naps, it's good to come up with a few enjoyable and easy activities like walking or cooking that you can do during your typical naptime. Avoid reading or watching TV during very low-energy times. If you absolutely must nap, you can experiment with an early catnap (try napping for 30 minutes or less during your afternoon dip in energy) and monitor whether that negatively impacts your nighttime sleep.

My Sleep Has Improved, but I Am Still Tired

Many strategies described in this book, particularly sleep restriction therapy and stimulus control therapy, are likely to increase fatigue in the short-term. You may be spending less time in bed and have less opportunity for sleep in the early stages of SRT and SCT. However, as your sleep consolidates, lengthens, and deepens, you should begin to feel more rested. If your sleep has improved and your fatigue remains unchanged or is still impactful, it's possible that the fatigue is due to something else. First, take note of your substance use, including alcohol, caffeine, and other stimulants, and medications. Consider whether you are ingesting substances that may be keeping you from restorative sleep. Also consider whether a stressful situation or mental health condition is possibly impacting your energy level. Importantly, long-lasting fatigue can indicate another sleep disorder or another health or mental health condition. You should speak with your physician and discuss getting a comprehensive work-up that looks at both your sleep and your overall health.

My Sleep Has Not Improved

If this is the case, first consider whether you are fully practicing everything recommended in this book. It is not uncommon for someone to try a strategy partially, or for a limited period of time, and then stop if it seems like the strategy is not working. For example, someone might do stimulus control therapy thoroughly for a couple of weeks, then become less diligent about it due to a vacation, illness, or disappointment that they haven't seen improvements yet. That is okay, but it is very important to realize that this does not mean stimulus control (or CBT-I in general) won't work for you. Sometimes it takes many weeks for someone to see significant improvements. With few exceptions, it's often the combination of sleep hygiene and behavioral strategies, as well as cognitive strategies and mindfulness and relaxation techniques, practiced diligently over time that eventually lead to big improvements in the quality and quantity of sleep.

That doesn't mean you have to make every change at once. You can make changes one at a time, building your sleep habits over time as you are ready. It is a worthwhile endeavor to reread your initial sleep assessment to review your specific trouble areas, and reread your sleep plan to see if there are areas where you can increase your efforts.

If you have truly stuck to your comprehensive plan and you can't identify any other areas where you can make changes, then there are a couple things to consider. First, we've discussed it's important to rule out other sleep, medical, or mental health conditions that

SLEEP STUDIES

If you suspect you have a sleep disorder, your physician can help you decide whether you need an overnight sleep study, also known as a polysomnogram. Sleep studies are very useful for diagnosing sleep disorders such as obstructive sleep apnea, narcolepsy (a type of hypersomnia), sleep-related seizure disorders, sleep-walking, or other sleep behaviors. Other sleep disorders can be diagnosed without a sleep study using clinical interviews, questionnaires, and sleep diaries. Some symptoms that may cause your physician to order a sleep study include snoring, pauses in breathing or gasping for breath when asleep, or excessive daytime sleep-iness. An in-lab overnight sleep study typically involves an electroencephalogram (EEG) test, which uses electrodes and other sensors to record brain activity. Other data such as heart rate, blood pressure, eye movements, muscle tone, oxygen levels, and leg and body movements are also collected. The overnight sleep study may even use video recording so that any unusual or problematic behaviors can be documented. Your physician may also order a home sleep study to check for sleep apnea. The home study often involves monitoring your breathing and blood oxygen level. With both in-lab and home studies, the information from the sleep study is typically combined with data from your medical history and sleep history to make a diagnosis.

may be impacting your sleep. Second, consider your stress and anxiety levels. If one or both are high, it may be helpful to increase your focus on mindfulness, relaxation, and stress-management strategies. If you feel that your thoughts about sleep or fears about not sleeping are the most impactful, mindfulness and acceptance are your biggest allies.

GETTING SUPPORT

Humans are social animals. Accessing help, support, and encouragement from others can be extremely useful when attempting to make significant changes or coping with a stressful situation. You may want to join a support group for people with insomnia or work with a psychologist or psychotherapist trained in CBT-I who can help you make the necessary changes to build healthy sleep habits. Starting therapy with a psychologist or other trained mental health professional can also help with anxiety, depression, or other life stressors and mental health issues. For more information on mental health, review the "Other Conditions That May Impact Sleep" section in chapter 1 (page 8).

Some of the changes you are making may impact a partner, roommate, friends, or family members. You may need their cooperation or support to successfully make changes. If this is the case, assertive communication is key. Asking for help from friends and family members can be difficult for some of us. And hoping or assuming others will know exactly what we need typically doesn't work. Making specific requests is more likely to result in you getting what you want or need. So, if you need someone's help in sticking to your sleep routine, tell them exactly how they can support you. For example, maybe you and your partner used to like to watch a TV show together in bed, and you know it would be helpful to watch it earlier, in the living room, before your nightly wind-down routine. Helping those around you understand why you are making changes, how these changes will benefit your sleep, and the specific actions they can take to support you may improve your relationships and your sleep quality. Having these conversations is more likely to result in you getting the help you want. So, keep talking, asking, and listening.

I hope that working through the CBT-I program has resulted in more restorative sleep and that you feel confident in your ability to continue nurturing and building good sleep habits. Many of the things you have learned and started to practice are aligned with a healthy lifestyle. I encourage you to continue to prioritize your health by promoting sleep and allowing sleep to come to you.

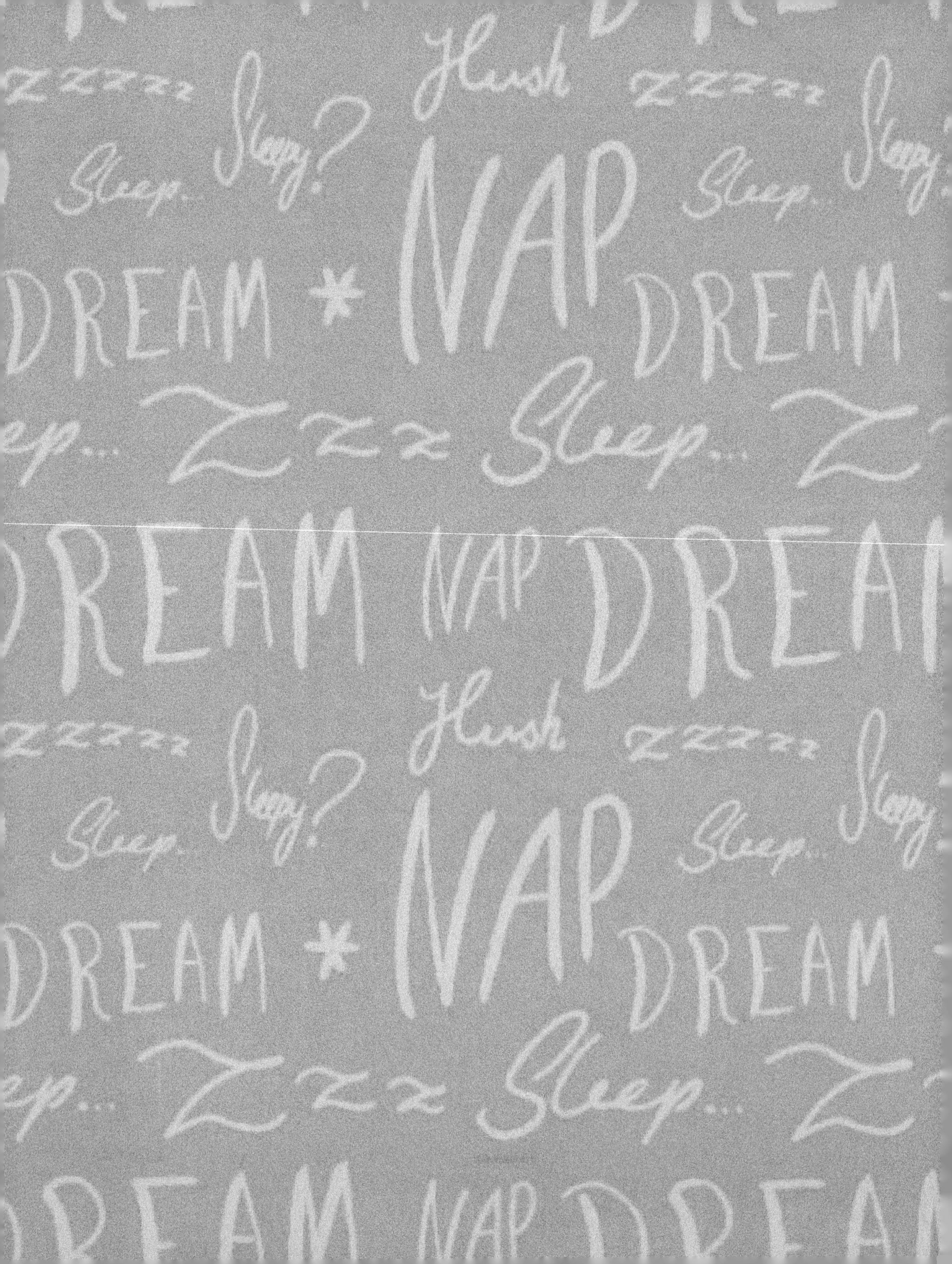
Hush
Zzzzzz
Sleepy?
Sleep...
NAP
DREAM
Zzz
Sleep...
DREAM
NAP
DREAM

BLANK WORKSHEETS AND FORMS

All worksheets and forms used in the book are included here for ease of use. You can find additional copies online at **www.CallistoMediaBooks.com/InsomniaWorkbook**.

THE SLEEP SELF-ASSESSMENT

INSTRUCTIONS: Please consider what your sleep and sleep habits have been like *for the past month.*

PART 1: SLEEP DURATION, EFFICIENCY, AND TIMING

During the last month:

1. On average, how many hours of sleep did you get each night? _____
2. a. On average, for how many hours were you in bed each night, both awake and asleep? _____
   b. Sleep Efficiency (Time Asleep ÷ Time in Bed) × 100 = _____%
3. On average, how long did it take you to fall asleep (Sleep Onset Latency)? _____
4. What time did you typically go to bed? _____
5. What time did you typically get up in the morning? _____

PART 2: SLEEP SYMPTOMS

Use the following scale for the questions below:

0   Never
1   Less than once a week
2   Once a week
3   2 to 3 times a week
4   4 or more times a week

During the past month, how often have you:

1. Had difficulty falling asleep? _____
2. Had difficulty staying asleep? _____
3. Woke up earlier than you wanted and weren't able to fall back to sleep quickly? _____
4. Felt your sleep quality was poor? _____
5. Felt fatigued during the day? _____
6. Canceled activities due to fatigue? _____
7. Had trouble staying awake during tasks like driving, eating, or socializing? _____

8. Relied on caffeine or other stimulants to get through the day? _____
9. Used a medication or substance to try and fall asleep? _____
   Please list what you took: _____
10. Worried about lack of sleep or not being able to sleep? _____
11. Thought about how difficult the next day would be due to lack of sleep? _____
12. Felt that an overactive mind was keeping you awake? _____
13. Felt too anxious, keyed up, or agitated to sleep? _____
14. Felt frustrated by not being able to sleep? _____
15. Had physical pain or discomfort that impacted your sleep? _____

Sleep Hygiene Factors

1. Had caffeine within 8 to 10 hours of bedtime? _____
2. Had alcohol within 3 hours of bedtime? _____
3. Napped? _____
4. Used screens while in bed (TV, phones, tablets, etc.)? _____
5. Watched TV or used other screens within one hour of bedtime? _____
6. Worked or engaged in other activities besides sleep or sex while in bed? _____
7. Felt your bedroom was too hot or cold, too noisy, or otherwise uncomfortable? _____
8. Felt that your sleep was disrupted by others (bedpartner, children, pets)? _____

Physical and Emotional Factors

1. Rate your stress level over the last month.
   (0 = no stress and 10 = extreme stress): _____
2. Rate your level of anxiety over the last month.
   (0 = no anxiety and 10 = extreme anxiety): _____
3. Rate your level of depression over the last month.
   (0 = no depression and 10 = extreme depression): _____
4. Rate your pain level over the last month.
   (0 = no pain and 10 = extreme pain): _____

DAILY SLEEP LOG*

Date: _____

PART 1: COMPLETE IN THE EVENING, BEFORE BED

How many caffeinated beverages? _____

Time of last caffeine? _____

How many alcoholic beverages? _____

Time of last alcohol? _____

Did you exercise? _____

Did you nap? _____

Medications/sleep aids? _____

How fatigued were you today? (0 = no fatigue to 10 = extreme fatigue) _____

PART 2: COMPLETE IN THE MORNING, UPON GETTING UP

What time did you get into bed? _____

What time was lights out? _____

What time did you fall asleep? _____

Sleep onset latency (time from lights out until asleep): _____

Number of awakenings (not including the final time you woke up): _____

How long for each? 1st: _____ 2nd: _____ 3rd: _____ 4th: _____ 5th: _____

Time of last awakening? _____

What time did you get out of bed? _____

Estimated total time asleep (TA)? _____

Total time in bed (TIB)? _____

Sleep efficiency? ([TA ÷ TIB] × 100) = _____%

Quality of sleep? (0 = poor to 10 = excellent) _____

Pain or discomfort? (0 = no pain to 10 = extreme pain) _____

Stress or Distress level? (0 = no distress to 10 = high distress) _____

Any in-bed activities? (watching TV, screens, work, reading, etc.)

_____

Other notes:

_____

* Adapted from "The 60-Second Sleep Diary" in *Say Goodnight to Insomnia*, by Gregg D. Jacobs.

WEEKLY SLEEP LOG SUMMARY

Week #: _____

Dates: _____

Average Sleep Onset Latency: _____

Average Estimated Time Asleep (TA): _____

Average Time in Bed (TIB): _____

Average Sleep Efficiency: ([TA ÷ TIB] × 100%) = _____%

Average number of awakenings: _____

Average fatigue: _____

Average quality of sleep: _____

Average stress/distress: _____

Average pain/discomfort: _____

What did you learn this week? Where have you made progress? What changes
were difficult? What was easier than expected? What were the roadblocks you
encountered, and how might you do it differently next week?

_____

_____

_____

_____

_____

_____

YOUR INDIVIDUALIZED SLEEP PLAN

RESOURCES

The following books, websites, and apps may be helpful supplements to your journey of building helpful sleep habits.

USEFUL WEBSITES

American Academy of Sleep Medicine's education page (SleepEducation.org).
This website provides information about healthy sleep and sleep disorders, as well as a list of AASM-accredited sleep centers in the United States.

American Sleep Association (sleepassociation.org).
This website provides information about insomnia and other sleep disorders, and available treatments.

The National Sleep Foundation (sleepfoundation.org).
This organization is dedicated to sleep education and advocacy and is a good resource for a range of sleep topics.

Psychology Today (psychologytoday.com).
This website has a wide range of psychology-related articles, as well as a therapist finder that can help you locate a mental health practitioner or support group close to you.

National Alliance on Mental Illness (NAMI.org).
This organization works to raise awareness and provide support and education about mental health to those who need it.

SLEEP BOOKS

Ehrnstrom, Colleen, and Alisha L. Brosse. *End the Insomnia Struggle: A Step-by-Step Guide to Help You Get to Sleep and Stay Asleep*. Oakland, CA: New Harbinger Publications, 2016.

Glovinsky, Paul, and Art Spielman. *The Insomnia Answer: A Personalized Program for Identifying and Overcoming the Three Types of Insomnia*. New York: TarcherPerigee, 2006.

Jacobs, Gregg D. *Say Good Night to Insomnia: The Six-Week, Drug-Free Program Developed at Harvard Medical School.* New York: Holt Paperbacks, 2009.

Walker, Matthew. *Why We Sleep: Unlocking the Power of Sleep and Dreams.* New York: Scribner, 2017.

MINDFULNESS, ACT, AND COMPASSION BOOKS

Hanh, Thich Nhat. *Peace Is Every Step: The Path of Mindfulness in Everyday Life.* New York: Bantam, 1991.

Hayes, Steven C., and Spencer Smith. *Get Out of Your Mind and into Your Life: The New Acceptance and Commitment Therapy.* Oakland, CA: New Harbinger Publications, 2005.

Kabat-Zinn, Jon. *Full Catastrophe Living: Using the Wisdom of Your Body and Mind to Face Stress, Pain, and Illness.* New York: Bantam, 2013.

———. *Wherever You Go, There You Are: Mindfulness Meditation in Everyday Life.* New York: Hatchette, 1994.

Neff, Kristen. *Self-Compassion: The Proven Power of Being Kind to Yourself.* New York: HarperCollins, 2015.

COGNITIVE BEHAVIORAL SELF-HELP BOOK

Burns, David D. *The Feeling Good Handbook.* New York: Plume, 1999.

MINDFULNESS AND RELAXATION APPS

10% Happier
Calm
Headspace
Insight Timer
Stop, Breathe & Think

REFERENCES

CHAPTER 1: INSOMNIA, BRIEFLY

American Psychiatric Association. *Diagnostic and Statistical Manual of Mental Disorders.* 5th ed. Arlington, VA: American Psychiatric Publishing, 2013.

Cappuccino, Francesco, Lanfranco D'Elia, Pasquale Strazzullo, and Michelle A. Miller. "Sleep Duration and All-Cause Mortality: A Systematic Review and Meta-analysis of Prospective Studies." *Sleep* 33, no. 5 (May 2010): 585–92.

Glovinsky, Paul, and Art Spielman. *The Insomnia Answer: A Personalized Program for Identifying and Overcoming the Three Types of Insomnia.* New York: TarcherPerigee, 2006.

Kecklund, Göran, and John Axelsson. "Health Consequences of Shift Work and Insufficient Sleep." *British Medical Journal* 355, no. 5210 (November 2016). doi:10.1136/bmj.i5210

Spira, Adam P., Lenis P. Chen-Edinboro, Mark Wu, and Kristine Yaffe. "Impact of Sleep on the Risk of Cognitive Decline and Dementia." *Current Opinion in Psychiatry* 27, no. 6 (November 2014): 478–83. doi:10.1097/YCO.0000000000000106

Smith, Michael T., and Jennifer A. Haythornthwaite. "How Do Sleep Disturbance and Chronic Pain Inter-relate? Insights from the Longitudinal and Cognitive-Behavioral Clinical Trials Literature." *Sleep Medicine Reviews* 8, no. 2 (April 2004): 119–32. doi:10.1016/S1087-0792(03)00044-3

Walker, Matthew. *Why We Sleep: Unlocking the Power of Sleep and Dreams.* New York: Scribner, 2017.

Williamson, Ann, and Feyer, Anne-Marie. "Moderate Sleep Deprivation Produces Impairments in Cognitive and Motor Performance Equivalent to Legally Prescribed Levels of Alcohol Intoxication." *Occupational and Environmental Medicine* 57, no. 10 (October 2000): 649–55. doi: 10.1136/oem.57.10.649

Van Dongen, Hans P., Greg Maislin, Janet M. Mullington, and David F. Dinges. "The Cumulative Cost of Additional Wakefulness: Dose-Response Effects on Neurobehavioral Functions and Sleep Physiology from Chronic Sleep Restriction and Total Sleep Deprivation." *Sleep* 26, no. 2 (March 2003): 117–126.

CHAPTER 2: SLEEP TECHNIQUES

Bent, Stephen, Amy M. Padula, Dan Moore, Michael Patterson, and W. Mehling. "Valerian for Sleep: A Systematic Review and Meta-analysis." *American Journal of Medicine* 119, no. 12 (December 2006): 1005–12. doi:10.1016/j.amjmed.2006.02.026

National Sleep Foundation's website (sleepfoundation.org)

Stahl, Stephen M. *Stahl's Essential Psychopharmacology Prescriber's Guide.* 6th ed. Cambridge: Cambridge University Press, 2017.

CHAPTER 3: BASELINE AND SLEEP ASSESSMENT

Ehrnstrom, Colleen, and Alisha L. Brosse. *End the Insomnia Struggle: A Step-by-Step Guide to Help You Get to Sleep and Stay Asleep.* Oakland, CA: New Harbinger Publications, 2016.

Jacobs, Gregg D. *Say Good Night to Insomnia: The Six-Week, Drug-Free Program Developed at Harvard Medical School.* New York: Holt Paperbacks, 2009.

WEEK 1: CHANGING YOUR SLEEP BEHAVIORS

Bootzin, Richard R., and Michael L. Perlis. "Stimulus Control Therapy." In *Behavioral Treatments for Sleep Disorders: A Comprehensive Primer of Behavioral Sleep Medicine Interventions.* Edited by Michael Perlis, Mark Aloia, and Brett Kuhn. London: Academic Press, 2011.

Glovinsky, Paul, and Art Spielman. *The Insomnia Answer: A Personalized Program for Identifying and Overcoming the Three Types of Insomnia.* New York: TarcherPerigee, 2006.

Morin, Charles M., Richard R. Bootzin, Danile J. Buysse, Jack D. Edinger, Colin A. Espie, and Kenneth L. Lichstein, "Psychological and Behavioral Treatment of Insomnia: Update of the Recent Evidence (1998–2004)." *Sleep* 29, no. 11 (November 2006): 1398–1114.

Walker, Matthew. *Why We Sleep: Unlocking the Power of Sleep and Dreams.* New York: Scribner, 2017.

WEEK 2: UNTHINKING YOUR WAY TO SLEEP

Burns, David D. *The Feeling Good Handbook.* New York: Plume, 1999.

Hayes, Steven C., and Spencer Smith. *Get Out of Your Mind and into Your Life: The New Acceptance and Commitment Therapy.* Oakland, CA: New Harbinger Publications, 2005.

Newman, Michelle G., and Thomas D. Borkovec. "Cognitive-Behavioural Therapy for Worry and Generalised Anxiety Disorder." In *Cognitive Behaviour Therapy: A Guide for the Practising Clinician.* Edited by Gregoris Simos. London: Taylor & Francis, 2002.

WEEK 3: RELAXING INTO SLEEP

Kabat-Zinn, Jon. *Full Catastrophe Living: Using the Wisdom of Your Body and Mind to Face Stress, Pain, and Illness.* New York: Bantam, 2013.

INDEX

ACKNOWLEDGMENTS

Thank you to Dr. Lindsay Whitman, Dr. Alyssa Lieb, Dr. Sherrie All, and Dr. Keith Cox for reviewing sections of the book and giving helpful feedback. I would also like to thank everyone at Callisto Media for their enthusiasm and guidance and for giving me the opportunity to write this book. Thank you to all the clients, friends, and family members who have shared their stories and sleep struggles with me. Finally, thank you to my husband, Tim, and my family and friends for their help and patience when writing took over early mornings, weekends, holidays, and multiple snow days. This project would not have been possible without your love and support.

ABOUT THE AUTHOR

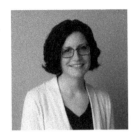

Sara Dittoe Barrett, PhD, is a licensed clinical psychologist who specializes in cognitive behavioral therapies and mindfulness for a wide range of presenting issues, particularly sleep, mood, anxiety disorders, obsessive-compulsive disorder, and chronic pain and illness. She works in private practice in Chicago, Illinois.

CPSIA information can be obtained
at www.ICGtesting.com
Printed in the USA
BVHW061732100619
550618BV00001B/2